LATE EFFECTS
OF TREATMENT
FOR CHILDHOOD
CANCER

CURRENT CLINICAL ONCOLOGY

Breast Cancer
B.J. Kennedy, M.D., *Editor*

Late Effects of Treatment for Childhood Cancer
Daniel M. Green, M.D., and Giulio J. D'Angio, M.D., *Editors*

LATE EFFECTS OF TREATMENT FOR CHILDHOOD CANCER

Editors

Daniel M. Green, M.D.
School of Medicine and Biomedical Sciences
State University of New York at Buffalo
Buffalo, New York

Giulio J. D'Angio, M.D.
Department of Radiation Oncology
Hospital of the University of Pennsylvania
Philadelphia, Pennsylvania

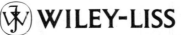

WILEY-LISS

A JOHN WILEY & SONS, INC., PUBLICATION
New York • Chichester • Brisbane • Toronto • Singapore

Address all Inquiries to the Publisher
Wiley-Liss, Inc., 605 Third Avenue, New York, NY 10158-0012

Copyright © 1992 Wiley-Liss, Inc.

Printed in the United States of America.

Library of Congress Cataloging-in-Publication Data

Late effects of treatment for childhood cancer / editors, Daniel M. Green, Giulio J. D'Angio.
    p. cm. — (Current clinical oncology)
  Based on the First International Conference on the Long-Term Complications of Treatment of Children and Adolescents for Cancer held in Buffalo, N.Y. from June 22–24, 1990.
  Includes index.
  ISBN 0-471-56167-3 (cloth). — ISBN 0-471-56166-5 (paper)
  1. Tumors in children—Treatment—Complications and sequelae--Congresses. I. Green, Daniel M. II. D'Angio, Giulio J. (Giulio John), 1922– . III. International Conference on the Long-Term Complications of Treatment of Children and Adolescents for Cancer (1st : 1990 : Buffalo, N.Y.) IV. Series.
  [DNLM: 1. Drug Therapy—adverse effects—congresses. 2. Neoplasms—in infancy & childhood—congresses. 3. Neoplasms--therapy—congresses. 4. Radiotherapy—adverse effects—congresses.
QZ 266 L3515 1990]
RC281.C4L38 1991
618.92'994—dc20
DNLM/DLC
for Library of Congress
      91-24273
      CIP

Contents

Contributors

Jeffrey Allen, M.D.
New York University Medical Center, New York, NY 10016 [55]

William L. Bigbee, Ph.D.
Biomedical Sciences Division, Lawrence Livermore National Laboratory, Livermore, CA 94550 [133]

Vilhelm A. Bohr, M.D.
Laboratory of Molecular Pharmacology, National Cancer Institute, NIH, Bethesda, MD 20892 [103]

Julianne Byrne, Ph.D.
Clinical Epidemiology Branch, National Cancer Institute, NIH, Bethesda, MD 20892 [113]

Mark A. Chesler, Ph.D.
Center for Research on Social Organization and Candlelighters' Childhood Cancer Foundation, University of Michigan, Ann Arbor, MI 48109 [151]

Judith M. Chessells, M.D.
Departments of Haematology and Growth and Development, The Institute of Child Health, London WC1, United Kingdom [89]

Peter E. Clayton, M.D.
Department of Endocrinology, Christie Hospital, Manchester M20 9BX, United Kingdom [71]

Elizabeth C. Crowne, M.R.C.P.
Department of Endocrinology, Christie Hospital, Manchester M20 9BX, United Kingdom [71]

Giulio J. D'Angio, M.D.
Department of Radiation Oncology, Hospital of the University of Pennsylvania, Philadelphia, PA 19104 [1]

Sarah S. Donaldson, M.D.
Department of Radiation Oncology, Stanford Medical Center, Stanford, CA 94305 [63]

Diane Fairclough, Dr.P.H.
Divisions of Psychology and Biostatistics, St. Jude Children's Research Hospital, Memphis, TN 38101 [31]

Wayne Furman, M.D.
St. Jude Children's Research Hospital, University of Tennessee College of Medicine, Memphis, TN 38101 [7]

Tracy A. Glauser, M.D.
Children's Hospital of Philadelphia and Children's National Medical Center, Philadelphia, PA 20010-2970 [41]

Stephen G. Grant, Ph.D.
Biomedical Sciences Division, Lawrence Livermore National Laboratory, Livermore, CA 94550 [121,133]

Janet R. Hancock, Ph.D.
Divisions of Psychology and Biostatistics, St. Jude Children's Research Hospital, Memphis, TN 38101 [31]

Daniel M. Hays, M.D.
Children's Hospital of Los Angeles, University of California School of Medicine, Los Angeles, CA 90054-0700 [171]

Barbara Hoffman, J.D.
Legal Counsel on the Employment Rights of Cancer Survivors and Adjunct Faculty, Seton Hall University, Cranbury, NJ 08512 [165]

Ronald H. Jensen, Ph.D.
Biomedical Sciences Division, Lawrence Livermore National Laboratory, Livermore, CA 94550 [133]

Edward Kovnar, M.D.
St. Jude Children's Research Hospital, University of Tennessee College of Medicine, Memphis, TN 38101 [7]

Larry Kun, M.D.
St. Jude Children's Research Hospital, University of Tennessee College of Medicine, Memphis, TN 38101 [7]

The numbers in brackets are the opening page numbers of the contributors' articles.

John Landsverk, Ph.D.
Children's Hospital of Los Angeles,
University of Southern California School of
Medicine, Los Angeles, CA 90054-0700 [171]

Richard G. Langlois, Ph.D.
Biomedical Sciences Division, Lawrence
Livermore National Laboratory, Livermore,
CA 94550 [133]

Shirley Lansky, M.D.
Illinois Cancer Council, Chicago, IL 60604
[159]

Timothy Lawther, B.A.
Center for Research on Social Organization
and Candlelighters' Childhood Cancer
Foundation, University of Michigan, Ann
Arbor, MI 48109 [151]

Alison D. Leiper, M.B.
Departments of Haematology and Growth
and Development, The Institute of Child
Health, London WC1, United Kingdom [89]

Lenore S. Levine, M.D.
St. Luke's–Roosevelt Hospital Center,
Columbia University College of Physicians
and Surgeons, New York, NY 10025 [55]

Marcy List, Ph.D.
Illinois Cancer Council, Chicago, IL 60604
[159]

Janine Maenza, M.D.
Columbia University College of Physicians
and Surgeons, New York, NY 10025 [55]

Mary McElwain, M.S.N.
Memorial Sloan–Kettering Cancer Center,
New York, NY 10021 [55]

Verna McHaney, M.C.D.
St. Jude Children's Research Hospital,
University of Tennessee College of
Medicine, Memphis, TN 38101 [7]

William Meyer, M.D.
St. Jude Children's Hospital, University of
Tennessee College of Medicine, Memphis,
TN 38101 [7]

Grace Powers Monaco, J.D.
Candlelighters' Childhood Cancer
Foundation, Washington, DC 20036 [179]

Raymond K. Mulhern, Ph.D.
Department of Psychology, St. Jude
Children's Research Hospital, Memphis, TN
38101 [23,31]

John J. Mulvihill, M.D.
Department of Human Genetics, University
of Pittsburgh, Pittsburgh, PA 15261 [113]

Sumit K. Nanda, M.D.
Eye Institute, Medical College of Wisconsin,
Milwaukee, WI 53226 [11]

Sharon E. Oberfield, M.D.
St. Luke's–Roosevelt Hospital Center,
Columbia University College of Physicians
and Surgeons, New York, NY 10025 [55]

Judith Ochs, M.D.
Department of Hematology–Oncology, St.
Jude Children's Research Hospital,
Memphis, TN 38101 [23]

Amanda L. Ogilvy-Stuart, M.R.C.P.
Department of Endocrinology, Christie
Hospital, Manchester M20 9BX, United
Kingdom [71]

Roger J. Packer, M.D.
Children's Hospital of Philadelphia and
Children's National Medical Center,
Philadelphia, PA 20010-2970 [41]

Vassilios Papadakis, M.D.
Memorial Sloan–Kettering Cancer Center,
New York, NY 10021 [55]

A. Pasos Papadimitriou, M.D.
Departments of Haematology and Growth
and Development, The Institute of Child
Health, London WC1, United Kingdom [89]

Jerilynn Radcliffe, Ph.D.
Children's Hospital of Philadelphia and
Children's National Medical Center,
Philadelphia, PA 20010-2970 [41]

Steven Ralston, M.D.
Columbia University College of Physicians
and Surgeons, New York, NY 10025 [55]

Chris Ritter-Sterr, M.S., R.N.
Illinois Cancer Council, Chicago, IL 60604
[159]

Kathleen Ruccione, R.N., M.P.H.
Children's Hospital of Los Angeles,
University of Southern California School of
Medicine, Los Angeles, CA 90054-0700 [171]

Jean E. Sanders, M.D.
Fred Hutchison Cancer Research Center,
Children's Hospital and Medical Center,
University of Washington School of
Medicine, Seattle, WA 98104 [95]

Andrew P. Schacha, M.D.
Ocular Oncology Service, Wilmer
Ophthalmological Institute, Johns Hopkins
University Hospital, Baltimore, MD 21205 **[11]**

Michael Schell, Ph.D.
St. Jude Children's Research Hospital,
University of Tennessee College of
Medicine, Memphis, TN 38101 **[7]**

Diana Schoonover, B.A.
Children's Hospital of Los Angeles,
University of Southern California School of
Medicine, Los Angeles, CA 90054-0700 **[171]**

Stephen M. Shalet, M.D.
Department of Endocrinology, Christie
Hospital, Manchester M20 93X, United
Kingdom **[71,81]**

Stuart E. Siegel, M.D.
Children's Hospital of Los Angeles,
University of Southern California School of
Medicine, Los Angeles, CA 90054-0700 **[171]**

Charles Sklar, M.D.
Department of Pediatrics, Memorial
Sloan-Kettering Cancer Center, New York,
NY 10021 **[49,55]**

Richard Stanhope, M.D.
Departments of Haematology and Growth
and Development, The Institute of Child
Health, London WC1, United Kingdom **[89]**

Russell Walker, M.D.
Memorial Sloan–Kettering Cancer Center,
New York, NY 10021 **[55]**

William H.B. Wallace, M.R.C.P.
Department of Endocrinology, Christie
Hospital, Manchester M20 9BX, United
Kingdom **[81]**

Margaret Weigers, M.A.
Center for Research on Social Organization
and Candlelighters' Childhood Cancer
Foundation, University of Michigan, Ann
Arbor, MI 48109 **[151]**

Susan L. Zilber, M.Phil.
Children's Hospital of Los Angeles,
University of Southern California School of
Medicine, Los Angeles, CA 90054-0700 **[171]**

Foreword

The number of newly diagnosed children with cancer in this country is small, relative to the overall cancer experience. There are about 6,000 cases each year. Fortunately, with the advances in treatment for childhood cancer during the past three decades, most of these children will be cured. Thus, each year there will be a cohort of children entering the group of an increasing number of childhood cancer survivors.

This book, which presents the results of an international conference held to discuss the long-term complications of treatment for cancer in children and adolescents, presents an in-depth look at an increasingly important problem. There are two major reasons why this topic is important to us. First, health professionals and the community at large should be aware of the special physical, psychological, and social considerations that may apply to a greater or lesser degree to the person who has survived childhood cancer. Second, by identifying late complications of significance, it may be possible to make correlations with specific components of therapy, in an effort to determine if some late complications might be avoided by modifying treatment, without sacrificing efficacy.

This book will be of great interest to any health professional who has responsibility to persons who have had cancer as children. The origins and nature of some of the clinical and psychological complications are well discussed. The consequences of treatment of cancer in children are obviously far different from the results of similar treatment in adults. Childhood is a time of physical growth and emotional development. These two features add entirely new dimensions to the usual side effects of cancer and its treatment that are experienced in adults. It is important for the health professional to realize that these effects can be lasting and persist long after childhood cancer has been cured. Emphasis in this book has also been placed on the equally important consideration of the social role of the cured cancer patient in the community. While rejoicing over the successes of the past three decades, the community is not always fully prepared to deal appropriately with the results of those successes—the survivors. This book provides the needed insights for health professionals to deal effectively with this growing segment of our population.

The book also contains discussions on the biological and clinical levels of the origins of these late complications. This aspect represents an important attempt to determine the degree to which these late complications can be avoided. There is an increasing fund of information about the molecular basis for some of the genetically determined childhood cancers. It is important that health professionals understand the genetic implications for some patients so that proper counseling can be provided. It must be realized that many of the studies represented in this book are based on children cured ten and twenty years ago. Current therapies are considerably different, and there must be ongoing studies for continuous evaluation of late complications of the treatment for childhood cancer. This book provides a cornerstone upon which future studies can be built.

Alvin M. Mauer, M.D.

Preface

The treatment of children and adolescents with cancer has become increasingly successful over the past 20 years. As a result, substantial numbers of survivors of cancer who were treated during childhood and adolescence now seek to complete their primary, secondary, and higher education; secure adequate employment; obtain adequate health and life insurance coverage; develop intimate relationships; and have children. Unfortunately, the treatment administered to eradicate the original cancer may produce side effects that interfere with the ability of a long-term survivor of childhood or adolescent cancer to achieve some or all of these goals.

The first International Conference on the Long-Term Complications of Treatment of Children and Adolescents for Cancer was held in Buffalo, New York, from June 22 to 24, 1990. The conference included 32 invited presentations from internationally recognized experts in five areas: 1) the effects of low-dose and high-dose radiation therapy on neuropsychological function, 2) the effects of low-dose and high-dose radiation therapy on pituitary function and growth, 3) the effects of radiation therapy and chemotherapy on gonadal function and reproductive outcome, 4) risk factors for the occurrence of second malignant tumors, and 5) psychosocial problems. The enthusiasm of the invited speakers and the conference participants indicated that the conference was timely and that survivors of childhood cancer provide fertile fields for further clinical investigation.

The present volume includes manuscripts summarizing the presentations given at the conference. The articles detail some of the specific problems encountered by long-term survivors following specific forms of treatment. The authors remind us that we are successfully treating today many children who previously would have died of cancer, but the present treatment are not without their costs. Some of those costs are just becoming known. This is because full assessment of possible iatrogenic complications must await completion of growth and development. Even then, latent damage may not be manifest for several years; eternal vigilance is therefore mandatory. The challenge in pediatric oncology remains clear: to strive for the cure and health of all children through the development of more effective yet less damaging treatment for our young patients.

The conference was co-sponsored by the Association for Research of Childhood Cancer, Inc.; Camp Good Days and Special Times, Inc.; Roswell Park Cancer Institute; National Cancer Institute; Beecham Laboratories, Inc.; and Lederle Laboratories, Inc.

The authors thank Mrs. Diane Piacente and Mrs. Gerri Ziolkowski for typing the manuscripts.

Daniel M. Green, M.D.
Giulio J. D'Angio, M.D.

An Overview and Historical Perspective of Late Effects of Treatment for Childhood Cancer

Giulio J. D'Angio M.D.

The long-term effects of the sometimes disabling and deforming surgical excisions for cancer have been known for centuries, and need hardly to be detailed. Radiation therapy became the first modality that could be added to surgery (or to replace it) in the management of cancer. Very early, pioneering therapists became aware of the deleterious effects of radiation on the developing organism. Indeed, the first radiobiological experiments were conducted by Perthes in 1903 [1]. He showed that the irradiated wings of chicks did not develop fully as did their nonirradiated counterparts. Very soon, Bergonie and Tribondeau [2], following a lead by Regaud, came to an important conclusion after irradiation of rat testes. They established that undifferentiated rapidly developing cells were more sensitive to radiation damage than those that were better differentiated and more slowly dividing.

EARLY EXPERIMENTS

The results of these early experiments had their obvious clinical connotations. The early workers in radiation therapy tried to exploit these observations for clinical benefit, while at the same time being wary of the damage so produced. In the former category were, for example, studies designed to straighten the curve in children with scoliosis [3]. Radium needles were implanted along the sides of vertebral bodies so as to slow growth in the adjacent apophyses and thus reduce the curvature. As the deleterious effects of radiation became clearer, however, the use of radiation therapy became more and more restricted to the management of malignant diseases. There was considerable attention paid even here to the growth disturbances resulting from irradiation. Wittenborg and his co-workers [4] at the Boston Children's Hospital noted the scoliosis that resulted from irradiation of the tumor bed in children treated for Wilms' tumors and neuroblastomas (Fig. 1). They reasoned that extending the field across the mid-line to encompass the entire vertebral body would result in symmetrical shortening. Thus, normal tissues not needed for the treatment of the basic conditions were irradiated in order to prevent a subsequent, delayed complication, namely, scoliosis. That technique has stood the test of time and is still used even today.

Remembering the work of Bergonie and Tribondeau, radiation therapists recognized that young children with malignant diseases would likely be more susceptible to damage, dose-for-dose. It therefore became commonplace to give age-adjusted doses of radiation therapy to children [5] (Table 1). This was done not in the belief that the tumor knew how old it was, as it

Late Effects of Treatment for Childhood Cancer, pages 1–6 © *1992 Wiley-Liss, Inc.*

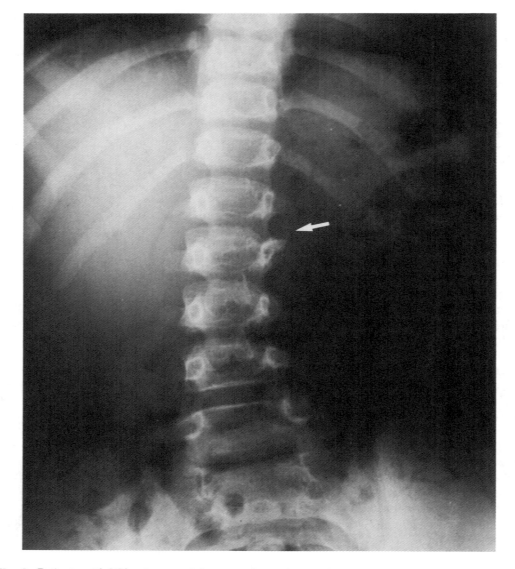

Fig. 1. Patient with Wilms' tumor eight years after radiation therapy. There is scoliosis of the lumbar column convex away from the irradiated flank. The whole vertebral body had not been included in the beam. Under these conditions, radiation to the ipsilateral portions of the vertebral apophyses shortens growth while the rest develops normally. A wedge-shaped deformity results. There is also an exostosis (osteochondroma) visible at the left border of L-2. The increased density adjacent to the pedicle represents the bony portion. The arrow points to calcification within the cartilagenous cap. This growth is among the more commonly seen benign tumors that develop in irradiated growing bones.

TABLE 1. Age-Adjusted Doses of Radiation Therapy Used in the First National Wilms' Tumor Study[a]

Age range (months)	Dose (cGy)
Newborn–18	1,800–2,400
19–30	2,400–3,000
31–40	3,000–3,500
41 +	3,500–4,000

[a]Modifications of this scheme are still in use for patients with anaplastic tumors Stages II–IV in NWTS-4, currently active.

were, but in recognition of the severe damage that would be produced if moderately high doses were given to an infant. It was an attempt to balance the consequences of perhaps underdosing the disease against the devastating late complications that would result from higher doses. The therapist thus accepted a possible higher risk of failure in babies as being a better choice than the certainty of a severely deformed survivor. As it happens, young children with neuroblastoma or with primary renal neoplasms, many of which are not Wilms' tumors, have a better outlook. They have therefore benefited from this approach over the years, even before the prognostic and histologic factors were understood and identified.

The survival rates for children with cancer were so poor for many decades that the late effects of irradiation could not be assessed; there were too few survivors [6] (Table 2). The advent of coordinated, multimodal therapy, including surgery, radiation therapy, and chemotherapy, improved survival rates. It then became evident that some tissues took longer to manifest late damage. These had been obscured because so many children died within months of treatment. A simple example is the failure to attain full growth at the time of the adolescent growth spurt [7]. Another is the fact that many years are needed before the

oncogenic potentials of irradiation are realized [8]. Both benign and malignant neoplasms can result (Fig. 1).

ISSUES IN CHEMOTHERAPY

These observations made by radiation therapists have their counterparts in chemotherapy. The issues there are far more complex because of the many different modes of action of the effective anticancer drugs. Attempts were made, nonetheless, to determine the long-term effects of chemotherapy on various organ systems. Taking a lead from Bergonie and Tribondeau, attention was soon paid to the gonad [9,10]. There was concern that the administration of chemotherapy might lead to sterility, teratogenesis, and genetic damage. Much of the initial animal work with chemotherapeutic agents was therefore turned to these problems.

It soon became evident, as new classes of drugs were synthesized or discovered, that each had its own spectrum of toxicities. Most shared myelosuppression, but pronounced organ-specific associated complications that are relatively drug-specific were soon identified. Examples are the bladder toxicity of cyclophosphamide and the pneuomonopathy associated with the nitrosoureas [11,12]. Even osteogenesis was affected by chemotherapy. Methotrexate, one of the most widely used drugs, disrupts protein anabolism, and osteopenias, fractures, and subluxa-

TABLE 2. Cancer Death Rates in Children Under 15 Years of Age by Decade[a]

Year	Death rate (million)
1950	80
1960	75
1970	55
1980	46

[a]Adapted from [6].

tions at the epiphyseal plates can result after prolonged usage [13].

Chemotherapy soon proved its value in the management of cancer in children, but the interaction between certain drugs and radiation therapy was unanticipated. The interplays of the anticancer antiobiotics and anthracyclines were soon identified through clinical observations. This emphasizes the role of the alert physician in defining the clinical pharmacology of any of these potent agents. It is a responsibility that cannot be left to laboratory colleagues; it must be shared with them. It was found that certain agents were capable of enhancing radiation reactions, and reactivating the latent radiation responses in treated tissues [14,15]. High doses of other chemotherapeutic agents, such as the alkylators, seem to have the same effect [16]. A new category of tissue damage came into being, namely, combined therapy toxicity. This realization had impact on the management decisions. It was recognized by oncologists dealing with children that local relapse could be a problem, but disseminated disease was more often the cause of death. Compromises were therefore reached with local treatments rather than with systemic chemotherapy. The doses of radiation therapy employed for such conditions as Ewing's tumor were reduced materially. It had been found that the ordinary doses in the 6,000–6,500-cGy range used for Ewing's tumor could not be tolerated by the bone and soft tissues when combined chemotherapy was added to the management [16].

Most of these observations were made within single institutions, but it was obvious that cooperative clinical trials would yield results more rapidly. The Late Effects Study Group (LESG) was formed for this purpose [8]. The cooperation of several leading investigators and institutions both in North America and Europe were enlisted in this endeavor. As the title of the group implies, data were collected from long-term survivors, and the effects on various organ systems studied. A major emphasis of the LESG has been on oncogenesis. The LESG has also maximized the usage of the collected data by making them available to epidemiologists, as well as running their own analyses [17,18]. This is a very fruitful approach to such complex issues. Now many of the cooperative study groups include long-term follow-up analyses among their objectives.

PROBLEMS OF CHILDHOOD SURVIVORS

One of the major problems in ascertaining late complications is the length of follow-up time needed, especially difficult when children are the subjects. As they get older, they mature from the pediatrician's office to those of relevant specialists, for example, gynecologists, internists, and the like [19]. It has been extremely difficult to interest those physicians who look after adults in the problems surrounding the child cured of cancer. Even medical oncologists remain aloof. They have many adult patients with very different tumor types and problems. The approaches used in pediatrics and the drugs employed are not familiar to the medical oncologist, and the result is a relative detachment from these particular issues. A solution appears to be one used in the armed forces for service people with rare diseases. Those afflicted with Hansen's disease, for example, carry their own medical dossier with them when they report to dispensaries for regular check-ups. The examining physician, who probably has never seen a Hansen's disease patient, is given a list of what needs to be done at that particular time. The same approach can be taken with adults who were cured of childhood cancer. Those who had irradiation near the thyroid gland, for example, can alert the physician to the need for thyroid function tests and for careful physical examination and imaging studies as needed to detect nodules. In short, the patient is the best conduit of information (and perhaps the most interested in seeing that the appropriate studies are accomplished) [20].

Important and sometimes neglected facets are the emotional and psychologic traumas sustained by both the family and the patient [21]. Parental fears and concerns at the time of diagnosis change as patient survival seems assured. They are replaced by worries about the adult the child will become. Will he/she be capable of leading a full life, undeformed, with intellect and sexual functions intact? Meanwhile, family life is disrupted; siblings suffer especially as parental attention is diverted [22]. Patients are obviously affected; the Damocles and Holocaust syndromes loom large for some. "Is the cancer going to come back?" "Why am I the survivor among so many others who died?"

Society is no less a participant in these dramas, albeit more detached. The benefits of decades of useful person-years gained when a child is cured are blunted as the taint of the original diagnosis hampers entry of the surviving adult into the work force [23]. Employability and insurability are reduced because industry reacts in misguided ways. Here is one arena where parents and health professionals can and must work together in educational efforts.

The need for continuing surveillance is certainly emphasized by the accumulating evidence of late cardiotoxicity in patients treated with Adriamycin [24,25]. Children and young adults who appear to be perfectly well nonetheless show signs of cardiac dysfunctions when studied carefully by appropriate examinations. Instances of sudden cardiac failure in women at the time of parturition are becoming more than the occasional anecdote.

Mechanisms must be set in place for the continuing, longitudinal study of cohorts of patients so that these untoward effects of successful treatment can be identified early. The cured cancer patient is now endemic in our society; it has been estimated that soon, if not now, 1 in every 1,000 twenty-year-old Americans will be a cured cancer patient [26]. Continuing follow-up of survivors by knowledgable, interested teams is obviously needed. These should include statisticians, epidemiologists, psychologists, nurses, and social workers, as well as clinical specialists.

Vigilance is essential if the blossoms of success in pediatric oncology are not to bear bitter fruit. Cure is not enough.

REFERENCES

1. Perthes G: Ueber den Einfluss der Roentgenstrahlen auf epithelial Gewebe insbensondere auf das Carcioma. Archiv Fuer Klinische Chirurgie 71:955–1000, 1903.
2. Bergonie J, Triboneau L: Interpretation de quelques resultats de la radiotherapie et essai de fixation d'une technique rationelle. Compt Rend Acad Sc Par 143:983–985, 1906.
3. Arkin A, Simon N, Siffert RS: Asymmetrical suppression of vertebral epiphyseal growth with ionizing radiation. Proc Soc Exper Biol Med 69:171–173, 1948.
4. Neuhauser EBD, Wittenborg MH, Berman CZ, Cohen J: Irradiation effects of roentgen therapy on the growing spine. Radiology 59:637–650, 1952.
5. D'Angio GJ, Evans AE, Breslow N, et al.: The treatment of Wilms' tumor: Results of the National Wilms' Tumor Study. Cancer 38:633–646, 1976.
6. Young JL, Ries LG, Silverberg E, Horm JW, Miller RW: Cancer incidence, survival and mortality for children under 15 years of age. Cancer 58:598–602, 1986.
7. Silber JH, Littman PS, Meadows AT: Stature loss following skeletal irradiation for childhood cancer. J Clin Oncol 8:304–312, 1990.
8. Mike V, Meadows, AT, D'Angio GJ: Incidence of second malignant neoplasms in children: results of an international study. Lancet 2:1326–1331, 1982.
9. Lentz RD, Bergstein J, Steffes MW, et al.: Postpubertal evaluation of gonadal function following cyclophosphamide therapy before and during puberty. J Pediatr 91:385–394, 1977.

10. Miller DG: Alkylating agents and human spermatogenesis. JAMA 217:1662–1665, 1971.

11. Gellman E, Kissane J, Frech R, Vietti T, McAlister W: Cyclophosphamide cystitis. J Can Assoc Radiol 20:99–101, 1969.

12. Durant JR, Norgard MJ, Murad TM, Bertolucci AA, Langord KH: Pulmonary toxicity associated with bis-chloroethyl nitrosourea (BCNU). Ann Intern Med 90:191–194, 1979.

13. Ragab AM, Frech RS, Vietti RJ: Osteoporotic fractures secondary to methotrexate therapy of acute leukemia in remission. Cancer 25:580–585, 1970.

14. D'Angio GJ, Farber S, Maddock CL: Potentiation of x-ray effects by actinomcyin-D. Radiology 73:175–177, 1959.

15. Donaldson SS, Glick J, Wilbur J: Adriamcyin activating a recall phenomenon after radiation therapy (Letter). Ann Inter Med 81:407–408, 1974.

16. Tefft M, Lattin PB, Jereb B, et al.: Acute and late effects on normal tissues following combined chemo- and radiotherapy for childhood rhabdomyosarcoma and Ewing's sarcoma. Cancer 37: 1201–1213, 1976.

17. Tucker MA, Meadows AT, Boice JD, et al.: Leukemia after therapy with alkylating agents for childhood cancer. J Nat Cancer Inst 78:459–464, 1987.

18. Tucker MA, D'Angio GJ, Boice JD, et al.: Bone sarcomas linked to radiotherapy and chemotherapy in children. N Engl J Med 317:588–593, 1987.

19. D'Angio GJ: The child cured of cancer: A problem for the internist. Sem Oncol 9:143–149, 1982.

20. Raymond CA: Childhood cancer improved survival rates can exact a price in late effects of therapy. Medical News and Perspectives. JAMA 260:3400–3405, 1988.

21. D'Angio GJ, Ross JW: The cured cancer patient: A new problem in attitudes and communication. In Proceedings of the American Cancer Society Third National Conference on Human Values and Cancer. Washington, DC: American Cancer Society, 1981, pp 45–59.

22. Schuler D, Bakos M, Zsambor C, et al.: Psychosocial problems in families of a child with cancer. Med Pediatr Oncol 13:173–179, 1985.

23. Meadows AT, McKee L, Kazak AE: Psychosocial status of young adult survivors of childhood cancer: A survey. Med Pediatr Oncol 17:466–470, 1989.

24. Hausdorf G, Morf G, Beron G, et al.: Long-term doxorubicin cardiotoxicity in childhood: Non-invasive evaluation of the contractile state and diastolic filling. Br Heart J 60:309–325, 1988.

25. Goorin AM, Chauvenet AR, Perez-Atayde AR, Cruz J, McKone R, Lipshultz SE: Initial congestive heart failure, six to ten years after doxorubicin chemotherapy for childhood cancer. J Pediatr 116:144–147, 1990.

26. Meadows AT, Krejmas NL, Belasco JB: The medical cost of cure: Sequelae in survivors of childhood cancer. In Van Eys J and Sullivan MP (eds): Status of the Curability of Childhood Cancers. New York: Raven Press, 1980, pp 263–276.

2

Effects of Radiation Therapy and Chemotherapy on Hearing

V. McHaney, M.C.D., E. Kovnar, M.D., W. Meyer, M.D., W. Furman, M.D., M. Schell, Ph.D., and L. Kun, M.D.

The hearing loss induced by cisplatin (CDDP) as a single agent is high frequency, bilaterally symmetrical, and irreversible. The deficit has been shown to be directly related to the dose of CDDP and inversely related to age. Less is known about possible synergistic ototoxic effects of CDDP with other anticancer agents. To identify factors that may potentiate ototoxicity, we compared the frequency of ototoxicity in patients receiving: 1) cranial irradiation given in different sequence, 2) CDDP and ifosfamide, or 3) standard CDDP followed by high-dose CDDP/etoposide (HDCDDP).

METHODS

Interaction of Cisplatin and Cranial Irradiation

To evaluate the interaction of cranial irradiation (CrRT) and CDDP, mean hearing thresholds were examined for 54 patients enrolled on three institutional brain tumor protocols between 1985 and 1989. Ages ranged from 2 3/12 to 20 3/12 years (mean 9 5/12 years). There were no significant age or sex differences between groups. Group I received cranial irradiation only. Group II received postoperative CDDP followed by CrRT, whereas Group III received CDDP as therapy for recurrent central nervous system (CNS) tumor after prior cranial irradiation. The interval be-

tween completion of CDDP (90 mg/m² × 4 doses) and initiation of CrRT was 3–4 weeks as defined by protocol in Group II. In Group III, the interval between CrRT and subsequent administration of CDDP (90 mg/m² × 4 doses) was 6–80 months (mean 32 months).

Interaction of Cisplatin and Other Chemotherapeutic Agents

To determine whether or not other drugs affect CDDP-induced hearing loss, we evaluated patients who had received both ifosfamide and CDDP. Patients enrolled on two successive osteosarcoma studies received equal doses of CDDP (100 mg/m² × 4 courses) and similar total dosages of doxorubicin and methotrexate. Forty-one patients enrolled on MIOS (POG 8107) represent the control group; serial audiograms were available for 17 patients. Nineteen patients enrolled on OS-86 (1986–1989) received CDDP following ifosfamide (1.6 g/m² × 5 for 5 cycles); all 19 patients received serial audiograms. The ages ranged from 4 to 23 7/12 years with no difference in mean age or age distribution in the two groups.

High-dose CDDP (HDCDDP) (40 mg/m² × 5 consecutive days) was administered to 20 children with neuroblastoma in relapse who had previously received CDDP at a conventional schedule of 90 mg/m²/dose. Total doses ranged from 90–1,220 mg/m² with a mean of 540 mg/m². Patients ranged in age from 2 4/12 to 18 9/12 years (mean 5 1/12 years) when first treated with CDDP. The interval between last CDDP and HDCDDP was 0–34 months (mean 10.2 months). Patients received 1–6 courses of HDCDDP (mean 4 courses). The cumulative dose of CDDP + HDCDDP ranged from 650–2,420 mg/m² (mean 1,250 mg/m²).

RESULTS

Interaction of CDDP and CrRT

In Group I, 23 patients receiving 5,400–6,000 cGy (centigray) CrRT alone had mean hearing thresholds at completion of CrRT within normal limits between 1,000 and 8,000 Hz. No patient had thresholds > 25 dB at 500–4,000 Hz. To determine the effect of sequencing CrRT and CDDP, hearing thresholds for patients who received CDDP prior to CrRT (Group II) were compared to patients with prior CrRT (Group III). Patients receiving CDDP after prior CrRT (Group III) had an 82% probability of having thresholds of 50 dB greater in the high-frequency range of 3,000 Hz or above after 360 mg/m² CDDP. The addition of subsequent CrRT in Group II did not increase the probability of further hearing loss in the speech range of 3,000 Hz or less. There was minimal increase in hearing loss following CrRT in those patients receiving preirradiation CDDP.

As shown in Figure 1, patients who received CDDP after prior CrRT (Group III) had mean hearing thresholds significantly worse than those tested after CDDP alone in Group II. Mean thresholds were stable following irradiation during follow-up intervals up to 56 months. Amplification has been recommended for 33% in Group II, compared to 80% of patients in Group III.

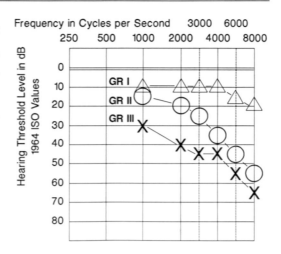

Fig. 1. Mean hearing thresholds for three groups of brain tumor patients. Group I (GRI) received cranial irradiation only (△—△); Group II (GRII) received CDDP (○—○) while Group III (GRIII) were administered cranial irradiation then delayed CDDP (X—X).

Interaction of Ifosfamide and CDDP

OS-86 patients showed normal hearing following three courses of ifosfamide prior to CDDP. Comparison of mean hearing threshholds showed that patients receiving ifosfamide prior to CDDP had significantly worse hearing than those patients receiving CDDP but no ifosfamide (Fig. 2). The resultant hearing loss may be more precipitous as compared to that seen with CDDP alone. Sixty-one percent of OS-86 patients exhibited a decrease of acuity of ≥40 dB from baseline or from one course of CDDP to the next. None of the patients receiving CDDP alone had shown a change of acuity of this magnitude with one course of CDDP. One patient with prior ifosfamide had a moderate sloping to severe hearing loss after only 100 mg/m²; the loss remained stable after 200-mg/m² dosage. Because of decreased hearing acuity at 2,000 Hz, the patient required binaural amplification. At cumulative CDDP dosage of 400 mg/m² following ifosfamide, amplification was recommended for almost 40% of patients due to hearing loss ≥30 dB at 3,000 Hz, as compared to 12% of MIOS patients.

Interaction of CDDP Plus High-Dose CDDP

Comparison of mean hearing thresholds at the last audiogram before high-dose CDDP versus the first audiogram after high-dose CDDP showed thresholds after high-dose CDDP were an average of 30–35 dB worse, especially in the speech frequencies of 500–3,000 Hz (Fig. 3). Two patients had been fit for amplification after CDDP alone because of hearing loss ≥40 dB at 2,000 Hz. After high-dose CDDP, an additional 16 patients (80%) reached this deficit level and required amplification.

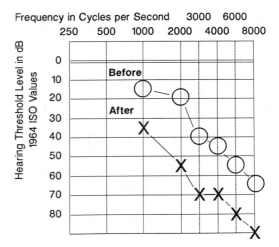

Fig. 3. Mean hearing thresholds for 19 patients after receiving their last course of CDDP but prior to high-dose CDDP (O—O) as compared to their mean hearing thresholds after administration of high-dose CDDP (X—X).

DISCUSSION

Cranial irradiation alone appears to have minimal ototoxic effect in the absence of subsequent chemotherapy. The combination of CrRT and CDDP has at least an additive dose-related effect and probably synergistic effect on hearing. This may be exacerbated in patients who receive CrRT prior to CDDP. The sequencing of CrRT and CDDP appears to be important, especially at 1,000–3,000 Hz, frequencies important for speech and language acquisition in younger children. CDDP following CrRT results in pronounced hearing deficits. The sequence of CDDP followed by CrRT results in substantially less ototoxicity. From the standpoint of ototoxicity, patients who appear to benefit from CrRT and CDDP are likely to experience less significant toxicity if given CDDP prior to irradiation. This may be of particular importance in young children with CNS tumors, in whom hearing loss may lead to further problems with communication and learning.

Ifosfamide, when given as a single agent, is not known to be ototoxic, but its use prior to CDDP appears to potentiate the ototoxicity of CDDP. The increased

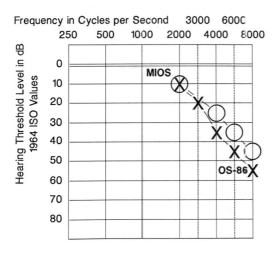

Fig. 2. Mean hearing thresholds for osteosarcoma patients who received identical cycles of CDDP only (O—O) as compared to those who received ifosfamide prior to CDDP (X—X).

ototoxicity is particularly relevant because ifosfamide and CDDP together are becoming regimens of choice in both pediatric and adult solid tumors.

Increased hearing loss in patients with neuroblastoma in relapse who received high-dose CDDP after previous CDDP is not unexpected. We are currently investigating whether the increased hearing loss is simply related to cumulative dose, or if other factors such as the interval between CDDP and high-dose CDDP, or schedule of administration, are involved.

CDDP, given alone or in combination with other antineoplastic agents, may lead to substantial hearing loss. Close audiologic monitoring is recommended in order to detect hearing loss at a time when intervention is necessary. This is particularly important in the very young child because the consonants that give intelligibility to speech are predominantly high-frequency sounds. Even with only a mild loss of hearing, a child will not properly be able to hear sounds that distinguish one word from another, that is, /ch/vs/sh/ (chop vs shop). Thus, even a minimal high-frequency hearing loss will have detrimental effects on the speech and language acquisition of preschool children, as well as the learning skills of school-age children. With the specificity of amplification available with current hearing aids, we advocate amplification and appropriate therapy for all young children showing ≥ 30 dB hearing loss at 2,000 or 3,000 Hz.

3

Ocular Complications Following Radiation Therapy to the Orbit

Sumit K. Nanda, M.D., and Andrew P. Schachat, M.D.

Ionizing radiation is an important therapeutic modality in the management of intraocular and orbital tumors in children. Small and medium-sized retinoblastomas can be treated with radioactive plaques and larger tumors with external beam irradiation. The use of radioactive plaques may be indicated when a solitary retinoblastoma is too large for either photocoagulation or cryotherapy. External beam irradiation is considered in retinoblastoma patients who have multiple tumors posterior to the equator, large symmertrical bilateral retinoblastomas, or smaller lesions inside the vascular arcades. Radiation has also been used to treat benign conditions affecting the orbital contents, and tumors growing in or near the orbit. These include rhabdomyosarcoma, metastases, sinus carcinomas with contiguous orbital involvement, "pseudotumor," thyroid ophthalmopathy, and lymphoma. Rhabdomyosarcomas are sensitive to both radiation and chemotherapy, and a combination therapeutic approach is currently employed. The eye may be exposed to radiation when prophylactic or therapeutic radiation is administered for central nervous system (CNS) neoplasms including pituitary tumors. Total body irradiation prior to bone marrow transplantation is an additional source of radiation to the eye. A host of ocular complications involving the anterior segment, posterior segment, or orbit may be encountered following radiation therapy. The following treatise will describe these ocular complications of radiation exposure.

LACRIMAL SYSTEM

Excess tearing (epiphora) may develop in approximately 20% of patients whose field of radiation includes the canalicular apparatus [1]. In several large series of eyelid basal cell epitheliomas treated by radiation therapy, epiphora developed after therapy in 5–10% of patients. The causes included: scarring of the canaliculi and puncta, ectropion of one punctum, failure of the lacrimal pump secondary to decreased eyelid mobility, and reflex lacrimation associated with ectropion, entropion, or conjunctival keratinization. As little as 1,800 cGy may cause canalicular stenosis. Intubation of the duct with a metal or silastic tube during and after radiation may prevent nasolacrimal duct obstruction [2]. Dacryocystorhinostomy, a procedure designed to reopen the lacrimal drainage system with the insertion of a silastic Jones tube, usually relieves the obstruction of the canalicular system. In many cases, the epiphora resolves spontaneously. This occurs because the radiation not only produces stenosis of the canalicular system, but also destroys some of the secretory glands of the lid and conjunctiva so that there is a reduction in the total quantity of tears produced. Thus, at some point, the impaired secretory mechanism and the damaged drainage system enter into compensatory equilibrium.

Radiation damage to the lacrimal gland may produce a "dry eye syndrome" (xerophthalmia). Karp et al. [3] reported a series of eight orbital exenteration specimens that demonstrated postirradiation involutional atrophy of the meibomian glands of the eyelids. These glands are responsible for the production of the lubricant component of the tear film. Stephens et al. [4] described an acute necrotizing dacryoadenitis occurring 24–48 hr after 250–2,000 cGy exposure to the ocular adnexa in primates. Acinar cells of major and accessory lacrimal glands and, to a lesser degree, lacrimal duct epithelium, showed degeneration and necrosis. These changes were increased in extent in proportion to the radiation dose. Reduced numbers of serous acini and decreased size of remaining acini indicate that atrophy of lacrimal glands can be recognized within two days after irradiation.

EYELIDS

Complications relating to eyelids and eyelashes include lid skin erythema, marked edema, lid margin epilation, entropion, ectropion, and fixed lower lid [2]. The eyelash is usually spared by megavoltage beam(s), so that it may remain at least partially intact even after maximum dose of 5,000–6,000 cGy deep to the lid. Acute reactions involving the lids and lashes are minimal and usually resolve within three months.

CONJUNCTIVA, CORNEA, SCLERA, AND IRIS

The acute reactions of the conjunctiva and sclera to high-dose irradiation are mild, transient, and well tolerated. Conjunctivitis, local telangiectasia, and keratin plaque formation in the palpebral conjunctiva have been reported [5].

The sclera is rarely affected by teletherapy since this avascular tissue is relatively radioresistant. Scleral necrosis may occasionally occur following use of radon seed, and tantalum wire implants, or other brachytherapy sources because of the very high local doses [6]. However, there are few indications for these treatments in children. Because retinoblastoma is relatively radiosensitive, the low doses administered by brachytherapy are usually well tolerated by the sclera.

The cornea is also a relatively avascular tissue and radiation-induced corneal changes result from disruption of mitotic activity in the epithelial and connective tissue layers. Clinical manifestations of injury are slow in appearing and require high doses. Severe corneal damage is characterized by inflammatory reaction of limbal vessels, punctate keratitis, corneal ulceration, thinning, and edema. Such damage is more likely to occur if secondary infection is present.

Anterior chamber complications are rare except after high dosages of radiation for intraocular tumors. Iridocyclitis may lead to extensive posterior synchiae formation. Iris neovascularization may occur and cause bleeding into the anterior chamber [5].

LENS

Cataracts are a frequent and visually threatening complication of radiation therapy to the eye. Radiation-induced cataracts have been demonstrated in a variety of experiments although the results vary with the X-ray doses employed and the subjects studied. Worgul et al. [7] produced lens opacities in frogs after an exposure of more than 1,000 cGy. He described the appearance of small, refractile dots in the equatorial subcapsular region of the lens. These dots increased in number and progressed to the posterior subcapsular region with time. Large vacuoles formed first in the posterior cortex and then in the anterior cortex. Cogan and Donaldson [8] found vacuoles along the posterior lens suture, granular opacities about the suture line, and paracentral, equatorial, and posterior subcapsular lesions following radiation exposure to rabbit eyes. The posterior subcapsular defect consisted of aberrant epithelial cells that migrated from the equator. These enlarged cells, known as the bladder cells of Wedl, had a pale-staining vesicular cytoplasm and relatively small nuclei.

Hayes and Fisher [9] reported the ultrastructural features of human lenses exposed to long-term, low-dose radiation. The anterior epithelial cells, germinal epithelium, and equatorial cortical fibers were altered. Feathery fibers, fiber liquefaction, and large, rounded membrane whorls were noted. The posterior cortical areas were also affected. Palva and Palkama [10] found vacuolated lens epithelial cells three days after irradiation. Edema occurred within a week and swelling and vacuolization of lens fibers with posterior subcapsular cataracts appeared after 30 days. At three months, the lenses had become completely opaque. In these experiments, cataracts developed within weeks to months; however, they may occur within hours after exposure to high doses of ionizing radiation [11].

There is disagreement regarding the minimum dose required for cataractogenesis following radiation. Some have reported that in experimental animals, cataract formation occurs near or above a dose of 1,000 cGy [7,11]. Richards et al. [12], however, found no effect at this dose. Increased damage [7,8,12,13] and decreased latency time have been observed as doses are increased. Worgul et al. [7] reported that younger subjects had a lower threshhold for cataractogenesis. Cogan and Donaldson [8] induced lens opacities in 10-week-old rabbits by administering 25

cGy or less, and Hockwin [14] obtained similar results in cows.

A review of the literature yields no obvious threshhold dose for humans, but analysis of data by Merriam and Focht [15] implies that some patients will develop cataracts after receiving 200 cGy in a single treatment, or 550 cGy when treatment is extended over more than three months. Although many patients may not develop cataracts after these exposures, adherence to these values as minimum doses would seem prudent. A single large dose seems to be more cataractogenic than a similar, fractionated total dose [16].

The mechanism of cataract formation following radiation therapy appears to be multifactorial. One hypothesis suggests that free radicals formed by the interaction of radiation with water interpose themselves between bonded atoms and break the bonds. Sulfhydryl-bearing proteins then reduce the free radical, thereby inactivating it. After donating an electron to the free radical, the remaining sulfur atoms bond to each other. Levels of these sulfhydryl-containing proteins have been reported to be decreased in the aging lens [17]. Infusions of glutathione [14,18,19], ascorbate [18,19], superoxide dismutase [19], and vitamin E [20] into lens preparations have demonstrated some protection against subsequently administered ionizing radiation. As these protective agents are lost, the risk of damage to the DNA of lens cells presumably rises.

Cells in the germinative zone of the lens are the most likely targets for radiation-induced damage to DNA. It is thought that ionizing radiation requires a threshhold number of "hits" on any one "target" of DNA to cause damage severe enough to affect mitosis. Low-level radiation can produce a slow accumulation of targets that have received nonlethal mutation-inducing damage that can lead to the production of abnormal proteins. These proteins, including those involved in suppression of free radical formation, become inactivated and allow further damage to DNA by free radicals. Ultimately, the protein damage accumulates, the distribution of proteins is altered, and a cataract forms [21].

In addition to the free radical damage to DNA, radiation may have a direct effect on other cell constituents, such as the lens proteins or membranes. It is estimated that a cell in the germinative zone requires almost three months to reach maturity [22]. Yet, cataracts have been produced in experimental models within weeks, and even within hours after exposure of the lens to large doses of radiation [11]. This evidence suggests that those cell constituents that have already formed may be damaged by radiation. A likely result of damage to lens cell membranes is a change in membrane permeability [18,23], with resulting shifts in cations [18,24]. The cations that have been implicated include sodium, potassium, and calcium.

MANAGEMENT OF ANTERIOR SEGMENT RADIATION INJURY

Anterior segment radiation injury is usually mild and, in general, treatable. When appropriate, shielding of anterior segment structures can avoid the problems completely. Complications are usually transient and often can be managed simply with ocular lubrication. In some cases of permanent lacrimal system damage, surgery to reopen stenosed drainage systems or chronic use of lubricants to supplement inadequate lacrimal gland function is required.

The probability of cataract formation rises with increasing dose. If visually significant cataract occurs, assuming that the optic nerve and retina are healthy (see below), cataract surgery is curative.

OPTIC NERVE

Damage to the optic nerve and the anterior visual pathways is a potentially blind-

ing complication of radiation therapy. It is more common when large doses of radiation are administered over a short time span. The total dose and fraction size are the key factors in determining the risk of optic neuropathy. Aristizabal et al. [25] found that 20% (5 of 26) of patients receiving more than 4,600 cGy developed optic nerve damage. In 106 patients treated with 220 cGy or less per fraction, there were only three complications (<3%) versus 12.5% (2 of 16) in those patients receiving over 220 cGy per increment. In the group of patients treated to 5,000 cGy at the rate of 250 cGy per fraction, 22% developed nervous tissue damage in contrast with 12.5% in those treated to the same total dose but at a rate of 200 cGy per increment. Parsons et al. [26] reported that the risk of injury correlated best with fraction size for patients who received more than 5,500 cGy. At 165–190 cGy per fraction, 6,000–7,300 cGy produced injuries in 8% (2 of 24) of patients. The risk within the same dose range was substantially greater (7 of 17, 41%) following daily doses greater than 195 cGy. Brown et al. [27] reported the development of an optic neuropathy after a mean dose of 12,500 cGy with brachytherapy compared to only 5,500 cGy after external beam therapy. At presumably "safe" doses of radiation therapy (<7,000 cGy delivered at <200 cGy/day), radiation-induced optic neuropathy has an increased incidence in patients with acidophilic adenomas [28], and in those receiving chemotherapy in combination with radiation therapy [29].

Radiation optic neuropathy is characterized acutely by hypermic disc swelling. It is often accompanied by peripapillary hemorrhages, hard exudates, subretinal fluid, and capillary nonperfusion (Fig. 1). Disc swelling usually abates after several weeks to months but often results in optic nerve pallor. Pathologic changes seen at autopsy or biopsy of the anterior visual

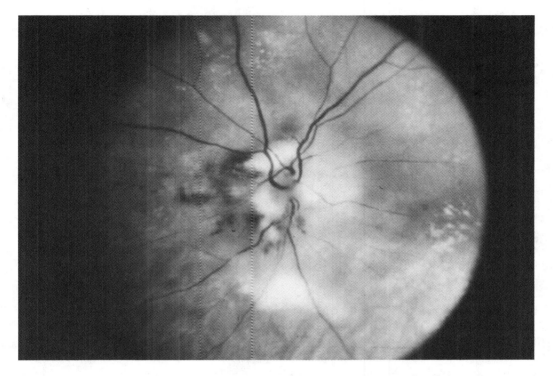

Fig. 1. Radiation optic neuropathy. Note the hemorrhages involving the optic disc, as well as cotton wool spots at the margin of the optic disc. The patient had received orbital radiation two years prior.

pathways have shown ischemic demyelination and an obliterative endarteritis [30]. The presumed mechanism of radiation-induced optic neuropathy is vascular damage with subsequent ischemia of the neural tissues.

The latency period from the termination of radiation therapy until the development of radiation-induced optic neuropathy appears to be shorter with brachytherapy (mean 12.6 months) than with external beam irradiation (mean 19.3 months) [27]. The overall prognosis for visual recovery after onset of optic neuropathy is generally poor [31]. However, Brown et al. [27] described two patients who had apparently "spontaneous" improvement of vision after mild visual loss resulting from radiation-induced optic neuropathy. Guy and Schatz [31] suggest

that hyperbaric oxygen therapy, administered within two weeks after the onset of radiation injury, may reduce the potential for severe visual loss. However, in a recent report by Roden et al. [32], 13 patients treated with hyperbaric oxygen and corticosteroids after delayed radiation injury to the optic nerves showed no visual improvement.

Radiation toxicity to the oculomotor nerves is manifested by an ocular neuromyotonia syndrome described by Lessell et al. [33]. This syndrome is a paroxysmal monocular deviation resulting from spasm of eye muscles due to spontaneous discharges from the third, fourth, or sixth nerve axons. Lessell observed this rare disorder in four patients treated with radiation for tumors in the region of the sella turcica and cavervous sinus.

RETINA

Retinal vascular changes and their associated sequelae are a visually threatening complication of radiation therapy. Stallard [34] first described radiation retinopathy in 1933. He reported the presence of exudates, hemorrhages, retinal pigment epithelial changes, optic disc edema, and atrophy. These developed in patients treated with radon seeds for retinoblastoma and capillary hemangioma of the retina. Retinopathy is characterized by the late onset of slowly progressive microangiopathy. It may result in macular edema, capillary nonperfusion, retinal and disc neovascularization, vitreous hemorrhage, and traction retinal detachment (Fig. 2).

The first animal model was described by Irvine and Wood [35]. They irradiated monkeys with 3,000 cGy and then examined their clinical and histopathologic findings. Focal loss of capillary endothelial cells and pericytes was initially seen. As areas of capillary dropout became confluent, cotton wool spots appeared, and subsequently faded to produce areas of retinal capillary nonperfusion. Histopathologic studies showed that deep, small retinal vessels were involved at first; these changes were followed by involvement of larger vessels. Intraretinal neovascularization occurred but no preretinal or disc neovascularization was noted. After 2.5–3.5 years, the monkeys developed rubeosis iridis and neovascular glaucoma.

As suggested by Irvine's monkey model, the presumed mechanism of radiation damage to the retina involves a vascular insult with endothelial cell damage

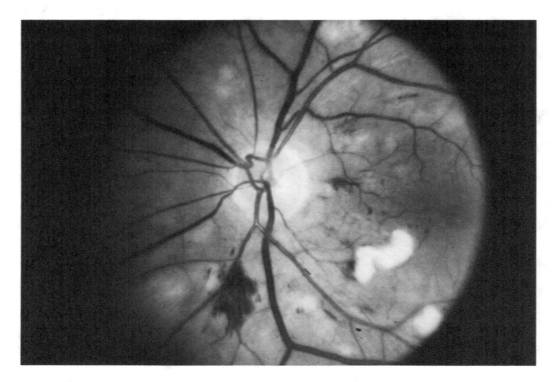

Fig. 2. Radiation retinopathy. The optic nerve appears normal but there are multiple retinal hemorrhages, microaneurysms, and cotton wool spots. The patient had received orbital radiation three years prior to presentation.

leading eventually to vaso-occlusive disease and its sequelae. Changes in vascular permeability produce edema and lipid. Histopathologic studies in humans revealed loss of capillary endothelial cells and pericytes, capillary and arteriolar occlusions, loss of ganglion cells (possibly secondary to neovascular glaucoma), and cystic changes in the outer plexiform and inner nuclear layers of the retina. Thickening of vessel walls, apparently from a deposition of fibrillary or hyaline material, has also been reported [36]. Myointimal proliferation may be present in larger vessels. In general, there appears to be preferential damage to inner retinal layers and the photoreceptors appear to be relatively resistant to radiation injury [36,37]. Animal studies show that rods may be damaged by doses of 2,000 cGy or more, while cones require doses exceeding 10,000 cGy before significant damage is seen [38].

The acute clinical retinal changes were described by Flick [39] in 1948 as featuring dilatation and engorgement of vessels, transient cotton wool spot formation and subsequent capillary nonperfusion, often involving the macula. Cystic macular edema may also be seen [40]. Following proton beam irradiation of 60 eyes with choroidal melanoma, 22% developed macular edema with an average follow-up of 18 months [41]. Late changes include retinal pigment epithelial cell (RPE) atrophy and generalized dispersion of the RPE leading to a "salt and pepper appearance." In the 1982 study by Brown et al. [42] involving 36 patients, 20 had received radioactive cobalt plaques (brachytherapy) for the treatment of intraocular tumors. The following clinical findings were noted: hard exudates (85%), microaneurysms (75%), intraretinal hemorrhages (65%), retinal vascular telangiectasia (35%), cotton wool spots (30%), and vascular sheathing (20%). The 16 patients who received external beam irradiation (teletherapy) showed hard exudates (38%), microan-

eurysms (81%), intraretinal hemorrhage (88%), retinal vascular telangiectasia (38%), cotton wool spots (38%), and vascular sheathing (25%). One of the 20 brachytherapy patients developed neovascularization, whereas two of 16 patients treated with external beam irradiation developed neovascularization of the disc (NVD), and five of 16 developed retinal neovascularization (NVE). Four of the 16 teletherapy patients developed neovascular glaucoma. The higher incidence of neovascular complications in patients treated with external beam irradiation is presumably due to the entire retinal area receiving the dose compared to only a localized area receiving radiation with brachytherapy. Although almost all patients in Gragoudas' and Brown's series were adults, the clinical findings are similar in children. The generalization that the larger the area of retina treated, the more severe the complications, still applies. In addition to the above microangiopathic changes, central retinal artery and vein occlusions have been reported following radiation therapy [43,44].

The microangiopathic changes usually become apparent six or more months after treatment, but sometimes may not appear until three years following treatment. In Brown's series, radiation retinopathy appeared 14.6 months (range 4–32) following brachytherapy and 18.7 months (range 7–36) following teletherapy.

The incidence of radiation retinopathy is dependent on both the total dose and the daily fraction size. The usual dose rate is 200–300 cGy/day, administered over a one- to two-month period for a total dose of 3,500–7,200 cGy [42]. Retinopathy may be seen after as little as 1,500 cGy of external beam irradiation [45], but usually 3,000–3,500 cGy are required before changes can be expected. One-half of the patients in two separate reports had retinal changes after 6,000 cGy; and after 7,000–8,000 cGy, 85–95% of the patients showed changes that were apparent within several months [2,46]. In another study of patients treated with radiation for sinus cancer, all who received more than 4,500–5,000 cGy showed retinal changes, although they usually did not develop visual loss. Mild reduction of vision was present following 6,500 cGy, however, and severe visual loss was seen in patients treated with 6,800 cGy or greater. The prevalence of retinopathy is higher at longer follow-up times. Brown et al. [42] observed that foveal damage occurred with a mean of 15,000 cGy (range 4,500–22,000 cGy) with cobalt plaque therapy. Those without foveal damage had received a mean dose to the fovea of only 5,000 cGy (range 3,500–9,000 cGy). Following external beam irradiation, how-

ever, the mean dose to the fovea that produced damage was 4,900 cGy (range 3,500–7,200 cGy). These data suggest that higher doses of brachytherapy are required to produce retinal damage than teletherapy.

The clinical findings of radiation retinopathy are similar to those of any retinal vascular disease that results in permeability or occlusive alterations. Fluorescein angiography may confirm the clinical diagnosis (Fig. 3). Areas of capillary nonperfusion are a consistent finding with the retinal capillaries affected earlier than the larger retinal vessels [42]. Hayreh [47] reviewed the angiographic findings, which included obliteration of retinal vessels, microaneurysm formation, telangiectasia, retinal neovascularization, cotton wool

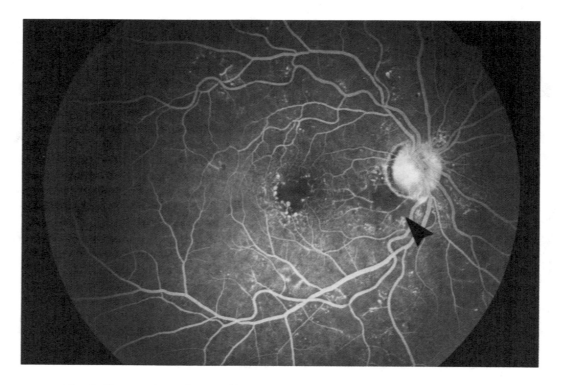

Fig. 3. Fluorescein angiogram. Note microaneurysmal dilatation of macular capillaries. There are multiple areas of capillary nonperfusion (arrow). The patient had received external beam radiation eight years before and first became symptomatic four years prior to the angiogram.

spots, hard exudates, retinal hemorrhage, cystoid macular edema, vascular sheath-ing and perivasculitis, optic disc edema, and disc neovascularization. The appear-ance of this entity may closely resemble that of diabetic retinopathy. Other entities in the differential diagnosis include multi-ple branch retinal artery obstructions, branch or central vein occlusions, and idi-opathic retinal telangiectasia. The diagno-sis should be suspected if the above clinical findings are present in association with a history of radiation therapy for any ocular neoplasm. Radiation retinopathy has also been described following orbital radiation for thyroid disease [48,49], or or-bital pseudotumor, and following intra-cranial radiation therapy for primary and CNS tumors [50]. It may also occur follow-ing radiation therapy for cancers of the paranasal sinuses [2] or the skin of the face and lids.

MANAGEMENT OF POSTERIOR SEGMENT DAMAGE

The management of the complications of radiation retinopathy consists of focal or grid laser treatment for macular edema and panretinal photocoagulation for neo-vascularization of the disc, retina, or angle. Gass [51] and Chee [52] reported successful focal treatment of macular exudates. Chaudhuri et al. [40] and Thompson et al. [53] described regression of proliferative changes following panret-inal ablation. In a recent study, Kinyoun et al. [54] successfully prevented further vis-ual loss in all five of the eyes they treated for macular edema. Three of the six eyes that received panretinal photocoagulation for proliferative retinopathy showed re-gression of neovascularization. The re-maining three progressed to develop dense vitreous hemorrhages requiring vit-rectomy. There is no available therapy for macular infarction.

Radiation retinopathy may produce vis-ual loss from foveal nonperfusion, macu-lar edema and exudates, vitreous hemor-rhage, neovascular glaucoma, and traction retinal detachment. The following three situations may exacerbate the retinopathy:

1. Patients with a preexisting microan-giopathy are prone to develop more severe changes. Diabetics show greater retino-pathic changes following lower doses of radiation than do nondiabetic patients [42,55].

2. Patients who receive certain chemo-therapeutic agents may show more severe changes even if the chemotherapy was not administered concomitantly [56]. In one report, patients who received 5-fluor-ouracil simultaneously with radiation therapy showed more frequent loss of vision.

3. Concomitant use of hyperbaric oxy-gen may also worsen radiation retino-pathy with severe retinopathy seen after only 3,600 cGy [57].

ORBIT

Complications involving the orbit con-sist of progressive contraction and fibrosis of the orbital soft tissues. Parsons et al. [26] reported spontaneous extrusion of or-bital implants, sutured in place after enucleation 1–5-months postoperatively. Radiation-induced contraction of the or-bital dead space was the likely cause of the implant extrusions. If external beam radi-ation is administered before growth is complete, as is usually the case with retinoblastoma and rhabdomyosarcoma, a characteristic sunken orbital appearance is seen.

SUMMARY

Radiation injury to the eye in children treated for retinoblastoma, rhabdomyo-sarcoma, and other malignant orbital tu-mors is usually severe and visually signifi-cant. However, the surgical approach to these tumors usually entails removal of the eyes, and the surgical results vis-a-vis survival often are no better than radiation. The use of radiation therapy despite its complications therefore seems appropriate. Because radiation damage is usually predictable, the patient and family should be warned of the potential complications. Most CNS tumors do not require high-dose orbital treatment, and ocular complications are relatively infrequent. The long-term effects of low-dose prophylactic CNS irradiation and total body irradiation are uncertain. It is to be hoped that these treatments will not lead to major long-term complications.

ACKNOWLEDGMENTS

This study was supported in part by a grant to A. P. Schachat from the American Cancer Society (CH 489-B).

REFERENCES

1. Call NB and Welham RAN: Epiphora after irradiation of medial eyelid tumors. Am J Ophthalmol 92:842–845, 1981.
2. Nakissa N et al.: Ocular and orbital complications following radiation therapy of paranasal sinus malignancies and review of literature. Cancer 51:980–986, 1983.
3. Karp LA, Streeter BW, Cogan DG: Radiation-induced atrophy of the meibomian glands. Arch Ophthalmol 97:147–155, 1979.
4. Stephens LC et al.: Acute radiation injury of ocular adnexa. Arch Ophthalmol 106:389–391, 1988.
5. Macfaul PA, Bedford MA: Ocular complications after therapeutic irradiation. Br J Ophthal 54:237–247, 1970.
6. Jones IS, Reese AB: Focal scleral necrosis: A late sequela of irradiation. Arch Ophthalmol 49:633, 1953.
7. Worgul BV et al.: Radiation cataractogenesis in the amphibian lens. Ophthalmic Res 14:73–82, 1982.
8. Cogan DG, Donaldson DD: Experimental radiation cataracts. I. Cataracts in the rabbit following single x-ray exposure. Arch Ophthalmol 45:508–522, 1951.
9. Hayes BP, Fisher RF: Influence of a prolonged period of low-dosage x-rays on the optic and ultrastructural appearance of cataract of the human lens. Br J Ophthalmol 63:457–464, 1979.
10. Palva M, Palkama A: Ultrastructural lens changes in x-ray induced cataract of the rat. Acta Ophthalmol 56:587–598, 1978.
11. Broglio TM, Worgul BV: Lens epithelium and radiation cataract. V. Observations on acid phosphatase and meriodional row nuclear fragmentation. Exp Eye Res 40:263–271, 1985.
12. Richards RD, Riley EF, Leinfelder PJ: Lens changes following x-irradiation of single and multiple quadrants. Am J Ophthalmol 42:44–50, 1956.
13. Rini FJ, Worgul BV, Merriam GRJ: Scanning electron microscopic analysis of radiation cataracts in rat lenses. I. X-radiation catartactogenesis as a function of dose. Ohthalmic Res 15:146–159, 1983.
14. Hockwin O: Early changes of lens metabolism after x-irradiation. Exp Eye Res 1:422–426, 1962.
15. Merriam GRJ, Focht EF: A clinical study of radiation cataracts and the relationship to dose. Am J Roentgenol 77:759–785, 1957.
16. Deeg HJ et al.: Cataracts after total body irradiation and marrow transplantation: A sparing effect of dose fractionzation. Int J Rad Oncol Biol Phys 10:957–964, 1984.
17. Giblin FJ, Chakravani B, Reddy WN: High molecular weight protein aggregates in x-ray induced cataract. Exp Eye Res 26:507–519, 1978.
18. Matsuda H, Giblin FJ, Reddy VN: The effect of x-irradiation on cation transport in rabbit lens. Exp Eye Res 33:253–265, 1981.
19. Srivastava VK, Richards RD, Varma SD: X-ray effects on lens DNA implications of superoxide (02). Acta Ophthalmol (Copenh) 61:860–868, 1983.
20. Ross WM et al.: Radiation cataract formation diminished by Vitamin E in rat lens in vitro. Exp Eye Res 36:645–653, 1983.
21. Lipman RM, Tripathy BJ, Tripathy RC: Cataracts induced by microwave and ionizing radiation. Surv Ophthalmol 33(3):200–210, 1988.
22. Tripathy RC, Tripathy BJ: Morphology of the normal, aging and cataractous human lens. I. Development and morphology of the adult and aging lens. Lens Research 1:1–42, 1983.
23. Lambert BW, Kinoshita JH: The effects of ionizing radiation on lens cation permeability, transport, and hydration. Invest Ophthalmol Vis Sci 6:624–634, 1967.
24. Hightower FR, Giblin FJ, Reddy VN: Changes in the distribution of lens calcium during development of x-ray cataract. Invest Ophthalmol Vis Sci 24:1188–1193, 1983.
25. Aristizabal S, Caldwell WL, Avila J: The relationship of time-dose fractionation factors to complications in the treatment of pituitary tu-

mors by irradiation. Int J Rad Oncol Biol Phys 2:667–673, 1977.

26. Parsons JT et al.: The effects of irradiation on the eye and optic nerve. Int J Rad Oncol Biol Phys 9(5):609–622, 1983.

27. Brown GC et al.: Radiation optic neuropathy. Ophthalmology 89(12):1489–1493, 1982.

28. Atkinson AB et al.: Progressive visual failure in acromegaly following external pituitary irradiation. Clin Endocrinol 10:469–479, 1979.

29. Fishman ML, Bean SC, Cogan DG: Optic atrophy following prophylactic chemotherapy and cranial irradiation for acute lymphocytic leukemia. Am J Ophthalmol 82:571–576, 1976.

30. Crompton MR, Layton DD: Delayed radionecrosis of the brain following therapeutic x-radiation to the pituitary. Brain 84:85–101, 1961.

31. Guy J, Schatz NJ: Hyperbaric oxygen in the treatment of radiation-induced optic neuropathy. Ophthalmology 93(8):1083–1088, 1986.

32. Roden D et al.: Delayed radiation injury to the retrobulbar optic nerves and chiasm. Ophthalmology 97(3):346–351, 1990.

33. Lessel S, Lessell IM, Rizzo JF: Ocular neuromyotonia after radiation therapy. Am J Ophthalmol 102:766–770, 1986.

34. Stallard HB: Radiant energy as (aA) a pathogenic and (b) a therapeutic agent in ophthalmic disorders. Br J Ophthalmol (Suppl 6):1–126, 1933.

35. Irvine AR, Wood IS: Radiation retinopathy as an experimental model for ischemia proliferative retinopathy and rubeosis iridis. Am J Ophthalmol 103:790–797, 1987.

36. Egbert PR et al.: Posterior ocular abnormalities after irradiation for retinoblastoma: A histopathologic study. Br J Ophthalmol 64:660–665, 1980.

37. Ross HS, Rosenberg S, Friedman AH: Delayed radiation necrosis of the optic nerve. Am J Ophthalmol 76:683–686, 1973.

38. Cibis PA, Noell WK, Eichel B: Ocular effects produced by high-intensity x-radiation. Arch Ophthalmol 53:651–663, 1955.

39. Flick JJ: Ocular lesions following the atomic bombing of Hiroshima and Nagasaki. Am J Ophthalmol 31:137–154, 1948.

40. Chaudhuri PR, Austin DJ, Rosenthal AR: Treatment of radiation retinopathy. Br J Ophthalmol 65:623–625, 1981.

41. Gragoudas ES et al.: Preliminary results of proton beam irradiation of macular and paramacular melanomas. Br J Ophthalmol 68:479–485, 1984.

42. Brown GC et al.: Radiation retinopathy. Ophthalmology 89:1494–1501, 1982.

43. Shukovsky IJ, Fletcher GH: Retinal and optic nerve complications in a high dose irradiation technique of ethmoid sinus and nasal cavity. Radiology 104:629–634, 1972.

44. Cogan DG: Lesions of the eye from radiant energy. JAMA 142:145–151, 1950.

45. Perrers-Raylor M, Brinkley D, Reynolds T: Choroido-retinal damage as a complication of radiotherapy. Acta Radiol Ther Phys Biol 3:431–440, 1965.

46. Merriam G Jr, Szechter A, Focht EF: The effects of ionizing radiations on the eye. Front Radiat Ther Oncol 6:346–385, 1972.

47. Hayreh SS: Post-radiation retinopathy: A fluorescence fundus antiographic study. Br J Ophthalmol 54:705–714, 1970.

48. Kinyoun JL et al.: Radiation retinopathy after orbital irradiation for Graves' ophthalmopathy. Arch Ophthalmol 102:1473–1476, 1984.

49. Kinyoun JL, Orcutt JC: Radiation retinopathy. JAMA 258:610–611, 1987.

50. Bagan SM, Hollenhirst RW: Radiation retinopathy after irradiation of intracranial lesions. Am J Ophthalmol 88:694–697, 1979.

51. Gass JDM: A fluorescein angiographic study of macular dysfunction secondary to retinal vascular disease. VI. X-irradiation, carotid artery occlusion, collagen vascular disease, and vitritis. Arch Ophthalmol 80:606–617, 1968.

52. Chee PHY: Radiation retinopathy. Am J Ophthalmol 66:860–865, 1968.

53. Thompson GM, Migdal CS, Whittle RJM: Radiation retinopathy following treatment of posterior nasal space carcinoma. Br J Ophthalmol 67:609–614, 1983.

54. Kinyoun JL, Chittum ME, Wells CG: Photocoagulation treatment of radiation retinopathy. Am J Ophthalmol 105:470–478, 1988.

55. Wara WM et al.: Radiation retinopathy. Int J Rad Oncol Biol Phys 5:81–83, 1979.

56. Chacko DE: Considerations in the diagnosis of radiation injury. JAMA 245:1255–1258, 1981.

57. Stanford MR: Retinopathy after irradiation and hyperbaric oxygen. J R. Soc Med 77:1041–1043, 1984.

Prospective Evaluation of Neuropsychological Function Following Cranial Irradiation or Intermediate Dose Methotrexate

Judith Ochs, M.D., and Raymond K. Mulhern, Ph.D.

As higher cure rates are sought in the subsets of children with acute lymphoblastic leukemia (ALL) who experience continued high relapse rates, choices for the majority of children among therapeutically equivalent regimens require consideration of acute and chronic toxicities [1–6]. A major identified area of concern is that of neuropsychologic outcome [7–31]. Retrospective studies linked 24-Gy cranial irradiation prophylaxis with adverse neuropsychologic sequelae, implying causation [10–19,22–28]. Today, the majority of children receive intrathecal (IT) prophylaxis [32], alone or in combination with methotrexate (MTX) infusions; [33] certain high-risk patients continue to receive radiation therapy, though at the lower dose of 18 Gy [34].

From June 1979 to December 1983, a randomized clinical trial at St. Jude Children's Research Hospital (SJCRH) was conducted to compare the efficacy of parenteral MTX (MTX group) and 18 Gy of cranial irradiation (RT group) as methods of central nervous system (CNS) prophylaxis [35]. A second study was designed to measure MTX pharmacokinetics and determine the degree of correlation with remission duration and outcome [36]. These two studies afforded a unique opportunity to prospectively measure and compare CNS changes associated with the two methods of prophylaxis and to determine if there was a positive correlation between adverse CNS sequelae and elevated plasma MTX levels.

STUDY DESIGN AND CONDUCT

Treatment

Eligibility criteria included an initial leukocyte count of $<100 \times 10^9$/L, no mediastinal mass, an absence of blast cells in cerebrospinal fluid, and blast cells lacking surface immunoglobulin and receptors for sheep red blood cells. Randomization was on the basis of age and initial leukocyte count.

Details of the treatment have been described elsewhere [35]. Table 1 compares the therapies for the two treatment groups.

Neuropsychologic Protocol

Within two weeks of diagnosis, 113 consecutive newly diagnosed children with ALL and their parents were asked to participate in the prospective neuropsychologic evaluations. Of the 108 who agreed, 49 patients remained in continuous complete remission for ≥4 years after elective therapy cessation and were fully evaluable; this total included 26 in the

Late Effects of Treatment for Childhood Cancer, pages 23–30 © 1992 Wiley-Liss, Inc.

TABLE 1. Comparison of Therapy Components for MTX and RT Groups

Therapy	MTX group	RT group
Induction	Same	Same
Cranial RT	None	18 Gy
ITMTX (12 mg/m²)		
Induction	Same	Same
CNS phase	weekly × 3	q 3 - 4 d × 5
Continuation	q 3 months × 10 (with IV MTX × 6)	~q 3 months × 10
Continuation duration	Same	Same
Continuation drugs	2	6
Intravenous MTX	1 g/m² × 15	None
Oral MTX	108 weeks	80 weeks
MTX exposure	Continuous	Intermittent
Total mg MTX/m²	168 mg IT MTX 2160 mg oral MTX 15,000 mg IV MTX	192 mg IT MTX 1600 mg oral MTX

MTX group and 23 patients in the RT group. The two cohorts were comparable with respect to age at diagnosis and final testing, intervals between first and last neuropsychological evaluation, initial leukocyte count, gender, and family socioeconomic status (data not shown) [37].

Neuropsychologic tests were scheduled to be administered as soon as possible after remission induction, at yearly intervals until cessation of therapy, and every other year during the next five years. Age-appropriate Wechsler tests were used to measure intelligence (IQ) [38–40], and Wide Range Achievement tests were used to measure academic achievement in reading (word recognition), spelling, and arithmetic [41]. A standardized Child Behavior Checklist was also obtained during the last few years of the study [42].

Full scale IQ tests and its two component parts (verbal IQ and performance IQ) can only be administered when the child is four years of age or older, and academic achievement tests can be given only when the child is in first grade or beyond. Due to young age, one-half of the children were not able to have their first evaluation done immediately after remission induction; all but two, however, had their initial evaluation while receiving antileukemic therapy.

Age-appropriate initial testing consisted of the Wechsler Preschool Scale for 14 patients, Primary Scale of Intelligence for 33 patients, and the Wechsler Intelligence Scale for Children-Revised (WISC-R) for two patients; the WISC-R was used for all final assessments and the Distractibility Index was calculated. Unless otherwise stated, IQ and academic achievement test score results in this report include only the initial and final neuropsychologic test scores.

Individual children were considered to have clinically important changes if the difference between their first and last scores was 15 points or more. This 15-point criterion was equal to one standard deviation from the test norms and was approximately three times the error of measurement of the test.

RESULTS

Treatment Results

Therapeutic results reported with a median four-year follow-up showed that approximately 67% of the MTX group patients and 56% of the RT group were in continuous complete clinical remission [43,44]. When patients were reclassified according to Rome Workshop Criteria [45], RT afforded greater protection than MTX in preventing CNS relapses among those classified as poor risk (91% ± 6% vs 78% ± 8%).

Group Score Decreases

Statistically significant changes were seen within, but not between, the MTX and RT groups when first and final IQ and academic achievement scores were compared [46]. The MTX group showed statistically significant decreases in their full scale IQ, verbal IQ, and arithmetic scores. The RT group also showed statistically significant decreases in their full scale, verbal IQ, and arithmetic achievement scores. With the exception of final arithmetic scores, the mean initial and final values for tests of intelligence or academic achievement were not significantly different from the mean values for a normative population.

Individual Score Decreases

In the MTX group, 18 (70%) of the 26 patients had one or more scores that decreased by 15 or more points (Figs. 1 and 2). Five patients (19%) had significant

enough declines in verbal and/or performance IQ scores to affect significant decreases in full scale IQ; two of the five patients also had significantly decreased achievement scores. Four patients had decreases in verbal or performance IQ scores accompanied by decreases in one or more academic achievement scores, and seven patients had significant decreases in one or more academic test scores. The frequency of reading and arithmetic score decreases was identical (27%); only three (12%) of 26 had decreased scores in spelling.

In the RT group, 13 (60%) of the 23 patients had one or more scores that decreased by 15 or more points. Five patients (21%) had significant enough declines in verbal or performance IQ scores to cause significant decreases in full scale IQ; two of the five also had significantly decreased achievement scores. Four patients had decreased performance or verbal IQ scores in addition to one or more decreased academic achievement scores, and two patients had one or more decreased achievement test scores. In the RT group, the frequency of significantly decreased scores was least in reading (8%), intermediate in spelling (16%), and most frequent in arithmetic (24%).

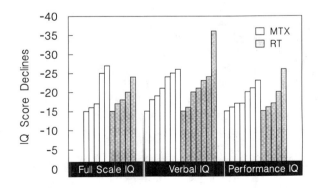

Fig. 1. Individual IQ score decreases from the initial to final evaluations for the MTX and RT groups. Each bar represents a single IQ score; the height of the bar indicates the degree of severity of the decrease. A single patient may be represented by one or more bars.

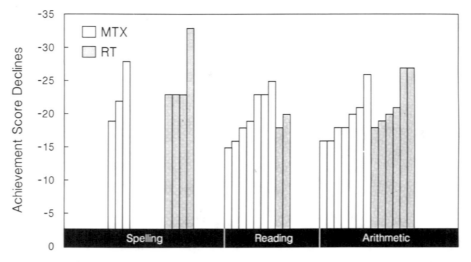

Fig. 2. Individual academic achievement score decreases from the initial to final evaluations for the MTX and RT groups. Each bar represents a single score; the height of the bar indicates the degree of severity of the decrease. A single patient may be represented by one or more bars.

Comparison of these results showed no significant difference in frequency or severity of decreased scores among individuals in the MTX and RT groups.

Individual Score Increases

We next examined individual score increases to determine if increased scores masked significant decreases when only group scores were examined.

In the MTX group, three patients (50%) had one or more clinically significantly increased scores (Figs. 3 and 4). Among these 13 patients, eight had both increased and decreased IQ or achievement scores, and five had only increased scores. In the entire group of 26 children, only five (19%) had no significantly decreased or increased IQ or achievement scores throughout the study's duration. In the RT group, 11 patients (48%) had one or more significantly increased scores. Among these 11 patients, four had both increased and decreased scores, and seven patients had increased scores only. Only three of 23 children (13%) had no significantly decreased or increased IQ or achievement score.

Patterns of Change

Although there was no discernible pattern of decreased or increased scores among individual patients, a pattern emerged that was common to both groups: significant frequency of clinically significant decreased full scale, verbal, and performance IQ scores and of scores in arithmetic. Over time, full scale IQ, verbal IQ, and arithmetic scores did not improve, but performance IQ, spelling, and reading did improve. The frequency of patients with significant decreases only (38%) was greater than the frequency of patients with both increased and decreased scores or with only increased scores. Overall, 24 or approximately one-half of the children showed one or more areas of improvement.

Behavior

On the Achenbach Child Behavior Checklist, only school performance was significantly low for age ($P < 0.01$). Hyperactivity and behavior problems were comparable with norms for the general population. Parents reported that 20

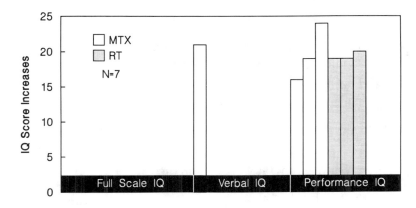

Fig. 3. Individual IQ score increases from the initial to final evaluations for the MTX and RT group. Each bar represents a single score; the height of the bar indicates the amount of increase. A single patient may be represented by one or more bars.

children repeated one or more grades, and 12 children received formal special educational assistance. There was no significant difference between the MTX and RT groups.

Associations and Correlations

Only two associations were found. Decreased verbal scores were associated with decreased reading scores ($P < 0.01$) and an age of less than four years in the MTX group was associated with decreased full scale IQ (5 of 15 vs 1 of 9 in the RT group, $P = 0.04$).

There were no significant associations or correlations between decreased IQ or achievement scores and treatment groups or elevated plasma MTX levels.

DISCUSSION

Examination of the findings in this prospective study comparing IQ and achievement scores in consecutive survivors of ALL randomized to two treatment

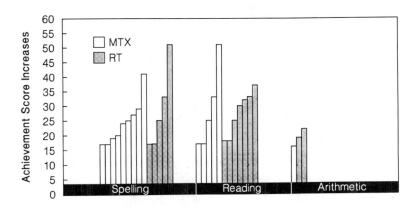

Fig. 4. Individual patient academic achievement score increases from the initial to final evaluations for the MTX and the RT groups. Each bar represents a single score; the height of the bar indicates the amount of increase. A single patient may be represented by one or more bars.

arms revealed four major, unanticipated findings.

Our first discovery was finding an almost identical frequency and degree of change in IQ and achievement scores regardless of the type of CNS prophylaxis. As compared to previous studies, the radiation dosage in this study was reduced by 25% (i.e., from 24 to 18 Gy). Due to the unacceptably high rate of CNS relapse using less aggressive MTX therapy in a previous clinical trial [33], MTX therapy in our study was intensified. Thus, the number of IT MTX injections and the duration of this therapy was increased (i.e., from 5 IT MTX injections over 2.5–3 weeks to 14 injections over 2.5 years). As a result, patients in our study received 10 times the amount of intravenous MTX and 5 times the amount of IT MTX, given over a period approximately 15 times longer. It is possible that reducing the irradiation dosage while intensifying parenteral methotrexate, produced comparable adverse neuropsychologic toxicity.

Second, we were also surprised by the high frequency of clinically significant decreases in IQ and achievement scores in individual patients over time. This type of data was obtained by use of a longitudinal design, which allowed us to use each patient as his/her own control. Sole use of mean group scores would had obscured the most meaningful information. The majority of children had a decrease in IQ and achievement scores. The decreased scores in order of their frequency were verbal IQ > mathematics > performance IQ > full scale IQ > reading ≫ spelling. Analysis of individual score decreases explains the high frequency of perceived learning problems reported by long-term ALL survivors and their families. Unfortunately, we were not able to determine the most efficient timing of evaluation for children who would eventually experience clinically significant decreases. Longitudinal data analysis revealed only a slow, steady, insignificant decrease in scores from one testing period to another.

The third unexpected finding occurred when we examined significantly increased scores. Not only did we find a substantial frequency of significantly increased scores, but these increases occurred almost exclusively in performance IQ, reading, and spelling achievement scores. Full scale IQ, verbal IQ, and mathematics achievement scores rarely improved. The finding that some children had increased scores implies that the neuropsychologic outcome in these children is more complex than previously thought.

The fourth unanticipated finding was the absence of any significant correlations between decreased IQ and academic scores and other variables, including the age at diagnosis, socioeconomic status, method of CNS prophylaxis, and serum MTX levels. Thus, we have been unable to find an effective, simple way to determine early in therapy which children will probably have adverse neuropsychologic sequelae.

Because the majority of children had one or more clinically significant decreases in IQ scores, achievement scores, or both, we were unable to determine any predictive factors. Optimal clinical management should include a neuropsychologic evaluation while on therapy and at least one evaluation after the patient has been off therapy 1 year or longer. The finding of increased achievement scores in one-half of the children is encouraging, however, and suggests that intervention can be successful.

ACKNOWLEDGMENTS

The author gratefully acknowledges the assistance of the medical editing department and the typing skills of Ms. Peggy Vandiveer. This work was supported by grants CA 21765 and CA 20180 from the

National Cancer Institute, and by the American Lebanese Syrian Associated Charities (ALSAC).

REFERENCES

1. Poplack DG, Reaman G: Acute lymphoblastic leukemia in childhood. Pediatr Clin North Am 35:903–932, 1988.
2. Niemeyer CM, Hitchcock-Bryan S, Sallan SE: Comparative analysis of treatment programs for childhood acute lymphoblastic leukemia. Semin Oncol 12:122–130, 1985.
3. Riehm H, Feickert H-J, Lampert F: Acute lymphoblastic leukemia. In Voute PA, Barrett A, Bloom J, et al. (eds): UICC Cancer in Children: Clinical Management, ed 2. Berlin: Springer-Verlag, 1986, pp 101–118.
4. Clavell LA, Gelber RD, Cohen HJ, Hitchcock-Bryan S, Cassady JR, Tarbell NJ, Blattner SR, Tantrahari R, Leavitt P, Sallan SE: Four-agent induction and intensive asparaginase therapy for treatment of childhood acute lymphoblastic leukemia. N Engl J Med 315:657–63, 1986.
5. Rivera GK, Kalwinsky DK, Rodman J, Kun L, Mirro J, Pui C-H, Abromowitch M, Ochs J, Furman W, Santana V, Hustu HO, Sandlund J, Crist WM: Current approaches to therapy for childhood lymphoblastic leukemia: St. Jude studies XI (1984–1988) and XII (1988). Modern Trends in Human Leukemia VIII. West Germany, 1988.
6. Blatt J, Bleyer WA: Late effects of childhood cancer and its treatment. In Pizzo PA, Poplack DG (eds): Principles and Practice of Pediatric Oncology. Philadelphia: Lippincott, 1989. pp 1003–1025.
7. Soni SS, Martin GW, Pitner SE, Duenas DA, Powazek M: Effects of CNS irradiation on neuropsychologic functioning in children with acute lymphoblastic leukemia. N Engl J Med 293:113–118, 1975.
8. Kirs PJ, Herman RM: Neuromotor and neuropsychological manifestations of 'total therapy' in children with ALL. Cancer Treat Rev 7:85–94, 1980.
9. Schuler D, Polcz A, Reversz T, Koos R, Bakers M, Gal N: Psychological late effects of leukemia in children and their prevention. Med Pediatr Oncol 9:191–194, 1981.
10. Moss HA, Nannis ED, Poplack DG: The effects of prophylactic treatment of the CNS on the intellectual functioning of children with ALL. Am J Med 71:47–52, 1981.
11. Meadows AT, Massari DJ, Fergusson J, Gordon J, Littman P, Moss K: Declines in IQ scores and cognitive dysfunction in children with ALL treated with cranial irradiation. Lancet ii:1015–1018, 1981.
12. Ivnik RJ, Colligen RC, Obetz SW, Smithson WA: Neuropsychological performance among children in remission from acute lymphocytic leukemia. J Develop Behav Pediatr 2:29–34, 1981.
13. Moehle KA, Berg RA, Chien LT, Lancaster W: Language related skills in children with acute lymphoblastic leukemia. J Devel Behav Pediatr 4:257–261, 1983.
14. Pavlosky S, Fisman N, Ariyaga K, Castann J, Chamules N, Leigvarda R, Moreno R: Neuropsychologic study in children with ALL: Two different CNS prevention therapies—cranial irradiation plus ITMTX versus ITMTX alone. Am J Pediatr Hematol Oncol 5:79–86, 1983.
15. Inati A, Sallan SE, Cassady JR, Hitchcock-Bryan S, Clavell LA, Belli JA, Sollee N: Efficacy and morbidity of 'prophylaxis' in children with acute lymphoblastic leukemia: eight years experience with cranial irradiation and intrathecal methotrexate. Blood 61:297–303, 1983.
16. Lansky SB, Cairns NV, Lansky LL, Cairns GF, Stephenson L, Garin G: Central nervous system prophylaxis: studies showing impairment in verbal skills and academic achievement. Am J Pediatr Hematol Oncol 6:183–190, 1984.
17. Pfefferbaum-Levine B, Copeland DR, Fletcher JM, Reid AL, Jaffe N, McKinnon WR: Neuropsychologic assessment of long term survivors of childhood leukemia. Am J Pediatr Hematol Oncol 6:123–128, 1984.
18. Rowland JH, Glidewell OJ, Sibley RF, Holland JC, Tuell R, Berman A, Brecher M, Harris M, Glicksman A, Forman E, Jones B, Cohen M, Duffner PS, Freeman A: Effects of different forms of central nervous system prophylaxis on neuropsychologic function in childhood leukemia. J Clin Oncol 2:1327–1335, 1984.
19. Whitt JK, Wells RJ, Laurie MM, Wilhelm CL, McMillan CW: Cranial radiation in childhood acute lymphocytic leukemia: neuropsychologic sequelae. Am J Dis Child 138:730–736, 1984.
20. Harten G, Stephani U, Henze G, Langerman HJ, Riehm AJ, Hanefeld F: Slight impairment of psychomotor skills in children after treatment of acute lymphoblastic leukemia. Eur J Pediatr 142:189–197, 1984.
21. Goff JR, Anderson HR, Cooper PF: Distractability and memory deficits in long term survivors of acute lymphoblastic leukemia. J Dev Behav Pediatr 1:158–163, 1980.
22. Eiser C: Effects of chronic illness on intellectual development. Arch Dis Child 55:766–770, 1980.

23. Eiser C: Intellectual abilities among survivors of childhood leukemia as a function of CNS irradiation. Arch Dis Child 53:391–395, 1978.
24. Eiser C, Lansdown R: Retrospective study of intellectual development in children treated for ALL. Arch Dis Child 52:525–527, 1977.
25. Berg RA, Ch'ien LT, Bowman P, Ochs J, Lancaster W, Goff JR, Anderson HR: The neuropsychological effects of ALL and its treatment—a three year report: intellectual functioning and academic achievement. Clin Neuropsych 5:9–13, 1983.
26. Copeland DR, Fletcher JM, Pfefferbaum-Levine B, Jaffe N, Ried H, Moor M: Neuropsychological sequelae of childhood cancer in long-term survivors. Pediatrics 75:745–753, 1985.
27. Jannoun L, Chessels JM: Long-term psychological effects of childhood leukemia and its treatment. Pediatr Hematol Oncol 4:293–308, 1987.
28. Tautman PD, Erickson C, Shaffer D, O'Connor PA, Sitary A, Carrera A, Schonfeld IS: Prediction of intellectual deficits in children with acute lymphoblastic leukemia. J Dev Behav Pediatr 9:122–128, 1988.
29. Schlieper AE, Esseltine DW, Tarshis MA: Cognitive function in long term survivors of childhood acute lymphoblastic leukemia. Pediatr Hematol Oncol 6:1–9, 1989.
30. Williams JM, Davis KA: Central nervous system prophylactic treatment for childhood leukemia: neuropsychologic outcome studies. Cancer Treat Rev 13:113–127, 1986.
31. Fletcher J, Copeland D: Neurobehavioral effects of central nervous system prophylactic treatment of cancer in children. J Clin Exp Neuropsych 10:495–538, 1988.
32. Sullivan MP, Chen T, Dyment PK, Hvizdala E, Steuber CP: Equivalence of intrathecal chemotherapy and radiotherapy as central nervous system prophylaxis in children with acute lymphatic leukemia. A Pediatric Oncology Group Study. Blood 60:948–958, 1982.
33. Freeman AI, Weinberg V, Brecher ML, Jones B, Glicksman AS, Sinks LF, Weil M, Pleuss H, Hananian J, Burgert EO Jr, Gilchrist GS, Nechles T, Harris M, Kung F, Patterson RB, Maurer H, Leventhal B, Chevalier L, Forman E, Holland JF: Comparison of intermediate-dose methotrexate with cranial irradiation for the post-induction treatment of acute lymphocytic leukemia in children. N Engl J Med 308:477–484, 1983.
34. Nesbit ME Jr, Sather HN, Robison LL, Ortega J, Littman PS, D'Angio EJ, Hammond GD: Presymptomatic central nervous system therapy in previously untreated childhood acute lymphoblastic leukemia: comparison of 1800 and 2400 rad. A report for the Children's Cancer Study Group. Lancet i:461–466, 1981.
35. Bowman WP, Ochs J, Pui C-H, Kalwinsky DK, Abromowitch M, Aur RJA, Rivera G, Simone JV: New directions of St. Jude total-therapy protocols: study X for standard-risk childhood acute lymphoblastic leukemia. In Murphy SB (ed): Leukemia Research: Advances in Cell Biology and Treatment. New York: Elsevier Biomedical, 1983, pp 203–211.
36. Evans WE, Crom WR, Stewart CF, Bowman WP, Chen CH, Abromowitch M, Simone JV: Methotrexate systemic clearance influences probability of relapse in children with standard-risk acute lymphocytic leukemia. Lancet i:359–362, 1984.
37. Hollingshead AB: Four Factor Index of Social Position. New Haven, CT, Yale University, 1975.
38. Wechsler D: Manual for the Wechsler Preschool and Primary Scale of Intelligence. San Antonio, The Psychological Corporation, 1967.
39. Wechsler D: Manual for the Wechsler Intelligence Scale for Children. San Antonio: The Psychological Corporation, 1949.
40. Wechsler D: Manual for the Wechsler Intelligence Scale for Children-Revised. New York: Psychological Corporation, 1974.
41. Jastak JF, Jastak S: The Wide Range Achievement Test Manual. Wilmington, DE: Jastak Associated, 1978.
42. Achenbach TM, Edelbrook C: The Child Behavior Checklist and Revised Child Behavior Profile. Burlington, VT: University of Vermont, Department of Psychiatry, 1983.
43. Abromowitch M, Ochs J, Pui C-H, Kalwinsky DK, Rivera G, Fairclough D, Look AT, Hustu H, Murphy SB, Williams WE, Dahl GV, Bowman WP: High dose methotrexate improves clinical outcome in children with acute lymphoblastic leukemia: St. Jude Total Therapy Study X. Med Pediatr Oncol 16:297–303, 1988.
44. Abromowitch M, Ochs J, Pui C-H, Fairclough D, Murphy SB, Rivera GK: Efficacy of high-dose methotrexate in childhood acute lymphocytic leukemia: analysis by contemporary risk classification. Blood 71:866–869, 1988.
45. Mastrangelo R, Poplack D, Bleyer A, Riccardi R, Sather H, D'Angio G: Report and recommendations of the Rome workshop concerning poor-prognosis ALL in children: biologic basis for staging, stratification and treatment. Med Pediatr Oncol 14:191–194, 1986.
46. Ochs J, Mulhern RK, Fairclough D, Parvey L, Whitaken JN, Mauer AM, Simone JV: Comparison of neuropsychologic functioning and clinical indicators of neurotoxicity in long term survivors of childhood leukemia given cranial irradiation or parenteral methotrexate: a prospective study. J Clin Oncol 9:145–151, 1991.

5

Methodological Issues in Studies of Neuropsychological Function After Treatment for Acute Lymphoblastic Leukemia

Raymond K. Mulhern, Ph.D., Janet R. Hancock, Ph.D., and Diane Fairclough, Dr.P.H.

As the number of long-term survivors of childhood malignancies has increased, so has the interest in describing their "quality of life." Objective and quantitative assessments of various components of quality of life such as performance status, satisfaction with self, and neuropsychological functioning have several important applications in pediatric oncology [1]. First, they define the economic, educational, and rehabilitative needs of long-term survivors, that will ultimately influence social programming at a national level. Second, studies of survivors can detect the sources of late sequelae of malignant disease and its treatment and, therefore, affect the development of contemporary treatment protocols. This information also assists the patient and his/her guardians in giving informed consent for treatment with a more complete knowledge of late complications. Finally, late effects studies provide the opportunity to investigate issues that may have general application beyond pediatric oncology, such as the relationship between age at onset of brain insult and the type and severity of subsequent neuropsychological deficits.

Neuropsychological studies of children treated for acute lymphoblastic leukemia (ALL) comprise a major segment of the late effects literature. This is at least in part because ALL is the most common malignancy of childhood, and has an expected 60–70% long-term survival rate in the past decade. Thus, relatively large numbers of patients with ALL are available for study. Early in the development of effective treatment for ALL, it became obvious that special attention to occult leukemia in the central nervous system (CNS) was necessary to insure maintenance of clinical remission [2]. Treatment with cranial irradiation, most often at a dose of 24 Gy, as well as intrathecal and systemic chemotherapy, was generally effective. Increasing concerns about the late toxicities to the CNS have now led to more selective CNS treatments, oftentimes with reduced doses or elimination of cranial irradiation for children with low risk of relapse in this site.

The present review will emphasize methodological problems that impede neuropsychological research of children previously treated for ALL. The actual findings of these studies is beyond the scope of this chapter; and the reader is referred to recent reviews by Williams and Davis [3] and Fletcher and Copeland [4]. Rather, we will attempt to make explicit

Late Effects of Treatment for Childhood Cancer, pages 31–39 © 1992 Wiley-Liss, Inc.

the primary causal variables of interest in this area, the process of choosing outcome measures, and critical factors in the design and implementation of neuropsychological studies of long-term survivors of ALL.

PRIMARY RISK FACTORS

Our review of the approximately 50 studies published on this topic reveals surprising consistency among the potential causal variables analyzed. These are 1) the patient's age at the time of CNS treatment; 2) the presence or absence of cranial irradiation in CNS therapy and its dose, if given; and 3) the amount of time elapsed since completion of CNS treatment [5]. The results of neuroimaging studies such as computerized tomography (CT) and magnetic resonance imaging (MRI) are sometimes chosen as a method of assigning patients to groups for subsequent analysis of neuropsychological findings but are more often presented as an additional index of brain damage.

At first glance, the solutions to methodological problems may appear straightforward but several factors inhibit the design of studies that can unambiguously address the risk factors cited above. Perhaps the overriding barrier is that only rarely has an ALL clinical trial been specifically designed to accommodate neuropsychological testing, thus allowing only limited control over the neuropsychological variables of interest. The patient's age at treatment cannot be manipulated by the investigator. Furthermore, an otherwise ideal design for testing a neuropsychological hypothesis may conflict with conventionally accepted treatment methods. For example, one may wish to study the potential interaction of age with different doses of radiation therapy. Such a study should enlist consecutively diagnosed patients, stratified on the basis of age and then randomized to receive no irradiation, the test dose and standard dose irradia-

tion. At most treatment centers, however, patients who are infants could not easily be accepted into the standard dose group nor could patients with CNS leukemia at diagnosis be accepted into the group receiving no irradiation. The end result is that, at best, neuropsychologic studies are considered adjunctive to the treatment protocol and are spliced into the prespecified treatment program. However, when patients are not assigned to treatment groups with appropriate consideration to the neuropsychological questions, problems in the analysis and interpretation of the resulting data are almost inevitable.

One wants ideally to eliminate any source of error that would limit the ability to generalize neuropsychological findings. The single most important factor to consider in this regard is the possibility of sampling bias. Enrolling consecutive patients who are eligible for the neuropsychological studies or randomly selecting from eligible patients is preferred. It is generally difficult to demonstrate the absence of sampling bias in "convenience" samples. Those children with significant problems may be overrepresented among those referred or volunteering for participation. One should document in studies of long-term survivors the reasons that otherwise eligible patients do not participate, so that these can be compared to the exclusionary criteria of other investigators. Among long-term survivors of ALL, we recommend excluding the following patient groups unless they are to be analyzed separately:

1. Patients with premorbid neurodevelopmental disorders such as Down's syndrome and seizures. The inclusion of patients with preexisting CNS abnormalities will decrease the ability to detect change compared to an otherwise normal sample of children diagnosed with ALL by depressing the initial "baseline" value.

2. Patients with CNS leukemia at diagnosis. One cannot detect the neuropsychological significance of this presenting feature in the absence of therapy since these children typically receive more aggressive CNS therapy.

3. Patients with any form of relapse. Relapses usually result in more aggressive and more toxic therapies, creating significant physiological, as well as psychological differences, between these patients and those who remain in complete remission.

Other decisions regarding inclusion and exclusion criteria are less rigid but present the investigator with difficult choices. Can patients treated on the same protocol at different institutions be considered equivalent? The practice is probably acceptable if the circumstances of the neuropsychological testing and the instrumentation are equivalent. What about the equivalency of patients who were treated at the same institution on different protocols? This is a very difficult issue. Even if one is assured that the CNS therapies on these protocols are not significantly different, differences among systemic therapy approaches may also have a direct effect on the CNS (e.g., intravenous methotrexate) or influence other factors correlated with test performance (e.g., longer total length of treatment).

A related issue is what variables, besides those associated with the patient's CNS treatment, may impact on neuropsychological performance. Among normal children, those with nonmalignant chronic disease, and those with cancer, two factors are implicated: socioeconomic status and school absences [6–8]. Children from lower socioeconomic strata and those who miss more school days because of illness perform significantly more poorly on tests of achievement and intellect. Therefore, these factors should be built into the assessment process and included in analyses of the neuropsychological data.

WHAT IS THE QUESTION?

Many investigators of the neuropsychological status of long-term survivors of ALL do not appear to have well-formulated questions or hypotheses. This general design flaw sometimes results in a "shotgun" approach to neuropsychological assessments with potentially misdirected resources as a consequence. In contrast to a decade ago when descriptions of global quality of life were significant additions to the literature, more specific and hypothesis-oriented studies are now needed with this population. This is not meant to imply that further exploratory studies are not needed; however, these should also be highly focused. Several contemporary research questions, in addition to those mentioned earlier, are presented in Table 1.

The questions asked will largely determine the study design. A major decision is whether to study patients at a single point in time (e.g., long-term survivors) or whether to study patients longitudinally. Cross-sectional studies are less expensive, less labor intensive, and offer a more immediate response to the neuropsychological questions. However, they cannot assess the change in patient performance over time, which is a requirement for answering several important questions. Both designs are susceptible to potential problems with selection bias, which should be indexed by the percent of eligible patients who were actually assessed. Cross-sectional studies do have an important role in neuropsychological research in providing results of exploratory analyses. These then assist in the development of longitudinal studies, that allow assessment of individual patient performance changes over time. One is therefore more secure in attributing causal influences to certain

TABLE 1. Current Research Issues in Neuropsychological Studies of Children With ALL and Selected References

Research question	Illustrative references
• Are children who are younger at the time of CNS treatment at greater risk of neuropsychological impairment than older children?	[9–12]
• Is CNS treatment with cranial irradiation more neurotoxic than intrathecal and systemic chemotherapy?	[12–14]
• What is the temporal relationship between CNS therapy and the appearance of neuropsychological deficits?	[8,15,16]
• Are the neuropsychological deficits specific or generalized?	[9,17]
• How do the neuropsychological deficits correlate with CT or MRI findings?	[18]
• Is the severity of neuropsychological abnormalities related to the dose of cranial irradiation received?	[19]
• Are there psychological interventions that can minimize or remediate neuropsychological sequelae?	None known
• What is the ultimate impact of neuropsychological deficits in terms of education, occupation, personal-social adjustment, and so on?	None known

events (e.g., cranial irradiation) if the patient has been assessed before and after the event. Longitudinal studies are extremely expensive, however. In order to illustrate this point, the study discussed by Dr. Ochs (see Chapter 4, this volume),

which spanned almost 10 years, enrolled 108 of 113 consecutively diagnosed patients with standard risk leukemia. Of those 108, 49 (45%) completed the study. Forty-eight (44%) relapsed, eight were excluded because of premorbid neurodevelopment or congenital conditions (7%), two refused to comply once enrolled, and one patient was removed from the therapeutic regiment because of hepatitis. If the aim of the study is to draw conclusions about the neuropsychological status only of long-term survivors, the data accrued on the excluded sample prior to their exclusion are discarded. All examinations in the above referenced study were provided without charge to patients and families. In situations where similar studies require the family to accept an additional financial burden, even if the examinations have clinical value, one can expect enrollment and compliance to be more problematic.

Another issue that depends on the question(s) asked by the study is whether or not external controls or comparison groups are needed, and if so, what their composition should be. If one is using standardized tests, the children comprising the test norms may serve as a "normal" comparison group but only if the investigator is certain that no systematic differences in socioeconomic and demographic characteristics exist between the groups. This comparison alone provides a weak argument for or against the presence of neuropsychological deficits. Patients may serve as their own controls in longitudinal studies that provide for serial evaluations over time. If the tests are corrected for normally expected improvements in performance with increasing age (e.g., most IQ tests), this provides a powerful method for evaluating neuropsychological changes. However, additional external comparison groups may be necessary to control for the nonspecific effects on chronic, life-threatening disease on personal-social and educational performance (e.g., children with cancer but no CNS therapy). Some studies have also used patient's siblings and schoolmates as controls but, in our opinion, these are most necessary in cross-sectional designs. In this case, the investigator usually assumes that the study group patients were not generally different from peers or siblings prior to CNS treatment. Any neuropsychological differences between the groups therefore implies that the study group has changed from premorbid status and assumes that the untreated comparison group has remained stable.

SENSITIVITY AND SPECIFICITY

Characteristics of the assessment measures are also important to consider when developing neuropsychological outcome studies. Standardized measures that are frequently used to assess levels of intellectual functioning include the Wechsler scales. These are composed of the Wechsler Adult Intelligence Scale-Revised (WAIS-R) for adults, the Wechsler Intelligence Scale for Children-Revised (WISC-R) for children aged 6–16 years, and the Wechsler Preschool and Primary Scale of Intelligence-Revised (WPPSI-R) for children aged 3½–7 years. The verbal, performance, and full scale IQ scores derived from these scales are normally distributed by age within the general population with a mean of 100 and a standardized deviation of 15 (see Fig. 1). From this distribution the percentage of age peers whose scores fall within a given range can be determined. For example, if a nine-year-old child obtains a verbal IQ score of 85, one can conclude that 84% of similarly age children scored *above* this level.

There is a certain amount of error as with any measurement in the assessment of an individual's IQ score. Some error variance is due to a test's less-than-perfect reliability. This is reflected by the test's standard error of measurement, which is determined by selecting the level of chance we are willing to accept that a person's true IQ score falls within a given range. For example, there is an 85% chance that a six-year-old's true full scale IQ score on the WISC-R falls within the

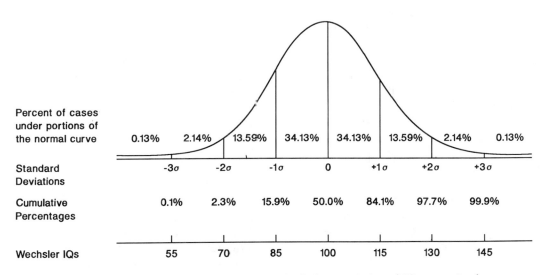

Percent of cases under portions of the normal curve	0.13%	2.14%	13.59%	34.13%	34.13%	13.59%	2.14%	0.13%
Standard Deviations		-3σ	-2σ	-1σ	0	$+1\sigma$	$+2\sigma$	$+3\sigma$
Cumulative Percentages		0.1%	2.3%	15.9%	50.0%	84.1%	97.7%	99.9%
Wechsler IQs		55	70	85	100	115	130	145

Fig. 1. Normative distribution and statistical characteristics of IQ scores in the general population.

range defined by the obtained IQ ±5 points, and a 95% chance that the same child's true score falls within the range of the obtained IQ ±7 points. The issue of test reliability is important when comparing an individual's IQ score at two points in time in order to detect change. If the first obtained IQ score was 85 for instance, and the second obtained IQ score was 87, each falls within the range of variance expected on the basis of chance fluctuations. For tests with lower reliability, there is a diminished ability to establish whether changes in IQ scores are actually a result of changes in ability level rather than chance fluctuations.

It can be seen that the importance of adequate standardization within the general population and well-defined reliability cannot be over-emphasized. Even with the better standardized psychological tests, these issues are of concern when interpreting the neuropsychological outcomes of treatments for ALL. The use of standardized instruments with novel populations for which no adequate norms have been established is a particular problem; and adoption of assessment devices without adequate established norms and unknown reliability appears to be an even greater one. When such measures are used, any interpretation of the resulting outcome data is questionable.

In general, psychological tests with the widest application, such as IQ and achievement tests, are better standardized. These measures, however, oftentimes afford only a global picture of the child's neuropsychological status. The more specific one becomes in choosing a test to measure a discrete neuropsychological function, the more difficult it may become to find adequate norms. For example, within one published series of test norms for the Halstead-Reitan Neuropsychological Battery, it is impossible for children to score more than 1.5 standard deviations below the mean for their age

group because this would yield a score below zero [20]. The investigator is advised to scrutinize test norms closely before including the test in the battery. Test score distributions that are highly skewed should be avoided.

EFFECT SIZE

The magnitude of the effect (effect size) expected in the study must be estimated when planning the design, the measures, and the analyses of neuropsychological data. The contrast between two groups at the same point in time (e.g., irradiated vs nonirradiated) will be the difference between the two group means divided by the standard deviation. If change in the performance of one group over time is being assessed, this will be the difference between the mean at time 1 and the mean at time 2 divided by the standard deviation (refer to Table 2). Consideration of these potential effect sizes is important in that it allows the investigator to calculate the sample size needed to detect such an effect and to balance this against institutional resources. Estimation of effect size also makes discrepancies between statistical and clinical significance more explicit. For example, with a sample size of 400 per group, a difference of 3 IQ points ($\alpha = 0.05$ and $\beta = 0.80$) could be detected reliably, but this difference is probably trivial in terms of its impact on the patient's functioning.

There are at least two ways that the psychological instrumentation can influence effect-size estimates. First, as discussed earlier, each test is associated with a known or unknown error of measurement that limits its sensitivity to difference between groups or changes over time. Difficulties in assessment increase substantially when small effect sizes approach the errors of measurement. Second, changes in tests or even changes in the version of the same test can introduce substantial er-

TABLE 2. Sample Size Computations at 80% Probability of Detecting a True Difference or Change[a]

Design	Effect size $\left[\dfrac{M_1 - M_2}{SD} \right]$	Equivalent IQ points	Required sample size/group		
			$r = 0.20$	$r = 0.50$	$r = 0.80$[b]
Contrasting	2.00	30	6		
groups	1.67	25	7		
	1.33	20	10		
	1.00	15	17		
	0.67	10	36		
	0.33	5	146		
Longitudinal	2.00	30	7	5	3
	1.67	25	8	5	4
	1.33	20	11	7	4
	1.00	15	18	10	6
	0.67	10	37	20	10
	0.33	5	147	74	31

[a]$\alpha = 0.05$, two-tailed tests of significance.
[b]Anticipated correlations among patient test scores at different points in time.

rors beyond those observed by repeated testing with the same test version over time. We have recently analyzed longitudinal data acquired over a nine-year period on children treated for leukemia. As children grew older, we were forced to measure the same neuropsychological factors with different tests or different versions of the same test. The statistical analysis revealed an approximate doubling of the expected error of measurement based upon repeated assessment with the same test, or the equivalent of 6–8 IQ points [8]. This becomes an even more important issue when one is seeking to detect relatively small changes in test performance. Tests with unknown psychometric reliability present special problems in estimating effect size.

STATISTICAL NOTES

The statistical analysis is a function of the question(s) to be answered by the study. These questions determine the study design (cross-sectional or longitudinal) and the psychological instruments,

which in turn determine the methods used in the statistical analysis. Psychological tests are often designed to identify children who have characteristics that are "unusual" relative to a reference population. Depending on the purpose of the instrument, the outcome measurement may be either categorical or continuous in nature. An instrument that identifies "problems" also classifies children into groups; thus, the outcome is categorical. A chi-square statistic may be used to test whether the frequency of "problems" is independent of treatment or patient characteristics. When multiple risk factors are considered simultaneously, techniques such as logistic regression or discriminant analysis can be used for categorical data.

The outcome measures from instruments that characterize the entire distribution of the study population are generally continuous. When continuous variables have a normal or symmetrical distribution, statistical tests such as Student's *t*-test, multiple regression or analysis of variance could be used to test for differences between groups or for associations of risk factors with differences in the outcome measures. When the distribution of continuous outcome measures is highly skewed, however, two approaches are possible. Either the data may be transformed using a function such as square-root, or a nonparametric statistical procedure may be used [21]. The skewed scores can be replaced by their corresponding ranks and the ranked scores can be analyzed by the appropriate parametric analysis [22]. When continuous outcomes are censored or a large proportion of the scores are tied, transformation and ranking are usually inadequate and the outcome measure will have to be treated as a categorical variable.

Studies with cross-sectional designs are generally uncomplicated to analyze and interpret when they are appropriate to the study question. Longitudinal designs with fixed points of measurement and no missing data can be analyzed using multivariate methods, but when longitudinal studies have random missing data and/or mistimed observations, the statistical analysis requires innovative techniques. One such approach assumes a mixed effects model [23]. If the missing data are nonrandom because they are related to the outcome that would have been observed, it is very unlikely that the statistical analysis can "fix" the bias in the study.

CONCLUDING REMARKS

Methodological problems present in studies of the neuropsychological status of long-term survivors of ALL are often a consequence of the design of the therapeutic protocol. Few, if any, front-line ALL treatment protocols will be designed to answer a neuropsychological question, especially when potential conflicts with accepted clinical practice arise (e.g., stratifying patients on the basis of age and then randomizing them to receive low dose,

high dose, or no cranial irradiation). As in other areas of clinical research, there may be interesting and important questions that cannot be addressed at all facilities treating patients with ALL. We recommend the following process in determining the feasibility and design of neuropsychological investigations in this area:

1. Carefully formulate questions and hypotheses.
2. Establish the sensitivity and specificity of tests.
3. Define the expected effect size.
4. Estimate sample size, statistical power, and compliance/attrition values.
5. Review institutional and collaborative group resources for patient accrual to relevant protocols and technical support.
6. Carefully define patient inclusion and exclusion criteria to avoid selection bias.
7. Insure adequate follow-up intervals.
8. Consider alternative control or comparison groups and cross-sectional versus longitudinal designs.
9. Design statistical analyses to address nonmedical covariates.

More recent neuropsychological studies have recognized the multivariate impact of ALL therapies on the performance of long-term survivors. The process of defining the relative contribution of potential risk factors will require increasing emphasis on select study samples and more complex statistical approaches. These are needed to compensate in part for diminished investigator control over some variables. Collaborative group studies (e.g., Pediatric Oncology Group or Children's Cancer Study Group) will be necessary in some instances to provide definitive answers to questions relating to the neuropsychological sequelae of the treatments given to children with ALL.

REFERENCES

1. Mulhern RK, Horowitz ME, Ochs J, et al.: Assessment of quality of life among pediatric patients with cancer. Psychological assessment. J Consult Clin Psychol 1:130–138, 1989.
2. Blyer WA, Poplack DG: Prophylaxis and treatment of CNS leukemia and other sanctuaries. Semin Oncol 12:131–148, 1985.
3. Williams JH, Davis KS: Neuropsychological effects of central nervous system prophylaxis for childhood leukemia. Cancer Treat Rev 13:113–127, 1986.
4. Fletcher JM, Copeland DR: Neurobehavioral effects of central nervous system prophylactic treatment of cancer in children. J Clin Exp Neuropsychol 10:495–538, 1988.
5. Ochs J, Mulhern RK: Late effects of antileukemic treatment. Pediatr Clin N Am 35:815–834, 1988.
6. Tautman PD, Erikson C, Shaffer D, O'Conner P, Sitarz Z, Correra A, Schonfeld IS: Prediction of intellectual deficits in children with acute lymphoblastic leukemia. J Dev Behav Pediatr 9:122–128, 1988.
7. Starr MC, Jarman FC: Academic achievement and its correlates in a community sample of chronically ill children (Abstract). Am J Dis Child 143:415, 1989.
8. Mulhern RK, Ochs J, Fairclough D: Neurobehavioral status of children surviving leukemia: A longitudinal analysis of patients randomized to receive low-dose irradiation or high dose chemotherapy. Personal communication.
9. Copeland DR, Fletcher JM, Pfefferbaum-Levine B, et al.: Neuropsychological sequelae of childhood cancer in long term survivors. Pediatrics 75:745–753, 1985.
10. Whitt JK, Wells RJ, Laurie MM, et al.: Cranial radiation in childhood acute lymphocytic leukemia: Neuropsychologic sequelae. Am J Dis Child 138:730–736, 1984.
11. Rowland JH, Glidewell OJ, Sibley RF, et al.: Effects of different forms of central nervous system prophylaxis on neuropsychological function in childhood leukemia. J Clin Oncol 2:1327–1335, 1984.
12. Ochs J, Mulhern RK, Fairclough D, et al.: Comparison of neuropsychologic functioning and clinical indicators of neurotoxicity in long-term

survivors of childhood leukemia given cranial irradiation or parenteral methotrexate: A prospective study. J Clin Oncol 9:145–151, 1991.
13. Moss HA, Nannis ED, Poplack DG: The effects of prophylactic treatment of the central nervous system on the intellectual functioning of children with acute lymphocytic leukemia. Am J Med 71:47–52, 1981.
14. Ivnik RJ, Colligen RC, Obetz SW, Smithson WA: Neuropsychological performance among children in remission from acute lymphocytic leukemia. Develop Behav Pediatr 2:29–34, 1981.
15. Jannoun L, Chessels JM: Long-term psychological effects of childhood leukemia and its treatment. Pediatr Hematol Oncol 4:293–308, 1987.
16. Robison LL, Nesbit ME, Sather HN, et al.: Factors associated with IQ scores in long-term survivors of childhood acute lymphoblastic leukemia. Am J Pediatr Hematol Oncol 6:115–121, 1984.
17. Mulhern RK, Wasserman A, Fairclough D, Ochs: Memory function in disease-free survivors of acute lymphocytic leukemia given central nervous system prophylaxis with or without 1800 cGy cranial irradiation. J Clin Oncol 6:351–320, 1988.
18. Brouwers P, Riccardi R, Fedio P, et al.: Long-term neuropsychologic sequelae of childhood leukemia: Correlation with CT scan abnormalities. J Pediatr 106:723–728, 1985.
19. Mulhern RK, Fairclough D, Ochs J: A prospective comparison of neuropsychological performance of children surviving leukemia who received 18 Gy, 24 Gy or no cranial irradiation. J Clin Oncol 9, 1991.
20. Knights RM, Norwood JA: Revised and smoothed normative data on the Neuropsychological Test Battery for Children. Ottawa, Canada, Carleton University, 1980.
21. Hollander MH, Wolfe DA (eds): Nonparametric Statistical Methods. New York: Wiley, 1973.
22. Conover WJ, Iman R: Rank transformations as a bridge between parametric and nonparametric statistics. Am Stat 3:124–133, 1981.
23. Vacek PM, Mickey RM, Bell DY: Application of a two-stage random effects model to longitudinal pulmonary data from sarcoidosis patients. State Med 8:189–200, 1989.

6

Prospective Evaluation of Neuropsychological Function in Children Treated for Medulloblastoma

Roger J. Packer, M.D., Jerilynn Radcliffe, Ph.D., and Tracy A. Glauser, M.D.

Improvement in the rate of survival for children with primary central nervous system (CNS) tumors has come extremely slowly [1]. In the last decade, however, progress has been made in some forms of childhood brain tumor [1–3]. Approximately one-half are malignant and most of the malignant tumors have a propensity to disseminate throughout the neural axis. It has been known for some time that malignant childhood brain tumors, such as medulloblastomas (MB) and possibly germinomas, are not truly localized diseases and require presymptomatic irradiation of the entire neural axis at diagnosis. This has resulted in an increase in the rate and duration of survival [1,3,4]. However, such extensive radiotherapy is potentially harmful to brain maturation and function [5].

As more children with MB survive free of progressive disease, the importance of their frequently permanent neurologic and cognitive sequelae has been magnified. The effects of the tumor, associated hydrocephalus, and perioperative complications all may result in neurologic or intellectual sequelae. Increased emphasis has been given in the past decade to the potentially damaging effects of treatment, especially the employment of presymptomatic craniospinal irradiation. The types of deficits these children have and the factors responsible for sequelae are still not fully elucidated.

HISTORICAL PROSPECTIVE

The first studies depicting cognitive deficits in children with MB appeared in the late 1960s and 1970s [6,7]. These reports utilized analyses of school performance or placement, the presence or absence of mental retardation, and global assessments of daily functioning. Bloom et al. [6] found that 82% (18 of 22) of survivors of MB had either minimal or no neurologic or cognitive disabilities. Jenkin [7] reported that 13% of 47 patients had either progressive mental retardation or significant school problems. Bouchard [8] recorded that only two of 18 children with medulloblastoma were mentally retarded or had learning difficulties at follow-up.

In the late 1970s and early 1980s, however, more detailed retrospective reports utilizing neuropsychometric measures of general intelligence painted a more dismal picture for survivors of MB. These reports were ushered in by a study from Raimondi and Tomita [9] who found that only five of 13 children surviving more than two years after diagnosis of MB were living completely normal lives. In this series, 33% of patients were retarded. Spunberg et al. [10], after studying 14 long-term survivors of a variety of tumors, found that 42% of the children had intelligence quotients falling in the retarded range. Specific learning problems were also found. In probably the most compelling retrospective study to date, Hirsh et al. [11] studied the cognitive abilities of 33 long-term survivors of primitive neuroectodermal tumors. All patients had received presymptomatic craniospinal irradiation and at least one-third had also received intrathecal methotrexate. This series utilized a control group of children with cerebellar astrocytomas. Of 26 patients studied, eight (31%) had IQ scores of less than 70 and 15 (58%) had IQ scores between 70 and 90. Emotional and behavioral disorders were also commonly found, occurring in 93% of the patients. Although some children with cerebellar astrocytomas had significant intellectual sequelae, a statistically significant difference was found between the children who had received radiation therapy and those who had not. Duffner et al. [12] reported similar pessimistic results in 10 long-term survivors with posterior fossa tumors who had undergone surgery, radiotherapy, and chemotherapy. Some of the 10 children also received intrathecal and intravenous methotrexate. Fifty percent (5 of 10) of children had IQ scores below 80 and all patients had either learning disabilities or mental retardation.

Somewhat at odds with these reports of severe damage in the majority of children was the retrospective experience at Children's Hospital of Philadelphia (CHOP). Of 24 long-term survivors of MB treated primarily with radiation (although some were given non-methotrexate chemotherapy) at CHOP between 1975 and 1984, the vast majority of children had psychometric scores that were in the normal range [13]. The median full scale IQ of 17 tested patients was 97. However, one-half of the children were in some type of special education placement and others had significant social and emotional problems. A major finding of this study, presented by Packer et al. [13], was that factors other than radiation significantly impacted on overall outcome. Children who presented with obtundation, or had significant perioperative complications, were more likely to suffer severe sequelae. Another factor that seemed to impact significantly on outcome was age at diagnosis. Lower overall full scale IQ (FSIQ) scores were associated with age of less than seven years at diagnosis. Other investigators also found that children who were younger at the time of diagnosis and treatment were more likely to have major learning disabilities [14,15].

Prospective Neurocognitive Studies in Children With Medulloblastoma

The results of the studies that utilized neurocognitive testing clearly showed that children with MB were at risk for developing neurocognitive sequelae. It also seemed clear that radiation played a significant role in cognitive dysfunction, but the impact of other factors was less well delineated. At the same time that these retrospective reviews were surfacing, the results of both retrospective and prospective studies in children with leukemia who had been treated with craniospinal radiation therapy became available [16]. Although often having serious methodological flaws, they showed that children with leukemia who had been given craniospinal irradiation had overall lower FSIQ scores than their counterparts who had not received whole brain irradiation. In 1981, Meadows et al. [16] documented a progressive decline in FSIQ in 11 patients who had been treated with both craniospinal radiation therapy and intrathecal methotrexate. This decline became statistically evident three years or more after treatment. The intellectual deterioration was most marked in children who were between the ages of two and five years at the time of diagnosis. This study, and others, highlighted the need for prospective evaluations for children with brain tumors.

At the present time, although many studies are underway, only a handful of studies have followed children long enough to draw even preliminary conclusions. Sixteen children with a variety of different brain tumors were followed by Duffner et al. [17]. Five had posterior fossa or pineal/suprasellar tumors and had received craniospinal irradiation. Three had MBs and two of these children had also been given methotrexate. Unlike their previous study, the authors found that only two of 16 patients had IQ scores in the retarded range. However, declines in IQ over time were seen and risk factors associated with falling IQs included younger age at the time of radiation and the use of adjuvant chemotherapy.

Ellenberg et al. [18] described a prospective study of 73 children with brain tumors treated over a three-year period at the Children's Hospital of Los Angeles. Forty-three had at least two sequential intellectual assessments, although not all had been given preradiation evaluations. All patients had some form of psychometric testing, but most received only some form of global testing such as the Bayley Scale for children under two, the McCarty Scale for children between two and six, and some variant of the WISC (Weschsler Intelligence Scale for Children) for children older than six years. Twenty-two of the 43 children with sequential tests had tumors of the fourth ventricle. Of these, 14 had received whole brain radiation—including 11 with MB. The age of the child at the time of treatment, and the use of whole brain radiation therapy, were associated with increased cognitive deficits. This was especially true in children who had received whole brain radiation and were under seven years of age at diagnosis. The report by Ellenberg et al. [18] is difficult to interpret. The overall follow-up was quite short and patients with tumors in many different areas of the brain were included in the study.

Beginning in January 1983, a study was begun at the CHOP prospectively evaluating all children with posterior fossa tumors who received craniospinal irradiation [19]. Children more than 18 months of age at diagnosis were eligible for study and results in only those who remained in continuous disease-free remission for the period of study were analyzed. A control group of children with cerebellar astrocytomas, who had tumors in a similar location as the children with MB, but who did not receive radiation therapy, were also psychometrically evaluated.

Children entered on this prospective study had detailed neuropsychological testing performed after surgery prior to radiotherapy, two to three months after completion of radiotherapy, and at one-year intervals, thereafter. The type of testing utilized varied with age. The test battery for children between 18 and 24 months of age was the Bayley Mental Scale of Infant Development, and for children between 24 and 36 months of age, the Stanford-Binet Intelligence Scale (form LM). Children more than five years old at the time of diagnosis had a more intensive neuropsychological battery. It measured global intelligence (WISC), but also assessed fine motor, visual–spatial, verbal fluency, language, memory, and auditory-attention abilities.

During the period of study, treatment was relatively uniform for children with MB. Patients who were between the ages of 18 months and 36 months of age at the time of diagnosis received a mean dose of 2,400 cGy of whole brain radiotherapy plus a local tumor "boost" of 2,400–2,600 cGy to the primary tumor site (total tumor dose: 4,800–5,000 cGy). Patients above 36 months of age at time of diagnosis received 3,600 cGy of whole brain radiotherapy plus a boost of 1,800–2,000 cGy to the tumor site (total tumor dose 5,400–5,600 cGy). In addition, the majority of children with MB received adjuvant chemotherapy consisting of cisplatin, CCNU, and vincristine. No intrathecal, oral, or intravenous methotrexate was used. During the first year of study, it became clear that it was difficult to test many of the children postoperatively, prior to the initiation of radiotherapy. For those children in whom testing was possible, results were compared to the immediate postradiotherapy study and the higher overall score was used as the child's baseline. In general, children tested higher two to three months postradiotherapy than they did after surgery prior to radiotherapy. The mean Full Scale Intelligence Quotient (FSIQ) for children (primarily those with MB) who went on to receive whole brain radiotherapy was 105. At year one, FSIQ fell to 97 and was down to 91 by year two. Smaller declines were observed in performance and verbal IQs. Compared with baseline testing, children demonstrated a statistically significant decline in FSIQ at year one (a decrease of 6.6) and at year two (a further decrease of 6.8). In addition, a marginal decline was identified in performance IQ at year two. Two years following treatment, two children had FSIQ scores below 70 and seven had FSIQ scores greater than 100.

This overall decline between baseline testing and performance at two years and full scale IQ and performance IQ scores inversely correlated with age. Two years following completion of craniospinal radiation, children who were seven years of age or less at diagnosis had a median decline of 25 points in full scale IQ to 82 as compared to 103 for older children.

No other parameters, including the occurrence of postoperative complications or the use of postirradiation chemotherapy, were significantly associated with overall intelligence or change in intelligence over time. Since the radiation dose varied little, it did not significantly correlate with outcome. The three youngest children in the study who received whole brain radiation therapy experienced the greatest decline in IQ scores. Even though these children were treated with a reduced dose of craniospinal radiation therapy (2,400 cGy), they had declines of 34, 36, and 37 points, respectively, in FSIQ between baseline and retesting two years later.

Children with cerebellar astrocytomas did not differ in intellectual parameters from those children with medulloblastomas at the time of diagnosis and did not show a decline in FSIQ over time. Thus, two years following diagnosis, there was a statistically significant difference in FSIQ and academic performance between the two groups.

Older children, who were evaluated for selective functional tests, showed a wide range of dysfunction. Mild to severe deficits in fine motor skills, especially in the dominant and to a lesser extent in the nondominant hand, were found both at time of baseline evaluation and two years following testing. However, there was no clear evidence that this function deteriorated over time. Significant visual-motor and visual-spatial impairments were infrequent. The number of children studied was small, but there was a trend for increasing memory deficits over time. Two years posttreatment, nearly one-half of the children performed below the normal range in list learning, while 64% had significant difficulties with immediate auditory recall.

The impact of treatment on school performance was marked. Eleven children who were to receive whole brain radiation therapy were in school at the time of diagnosis, and all were in a regular classroom. Two years after completion of radiation therapy, only six of the children remained at that level. All seven children, who were not yet in a regular classroom placement at the time of diagnosis because of young age, required special education placement when they began formal education. On the Wide Range Achievement Test, patients tended to score poorer in mathematical function than in reading or spelling. There was a significant decline between baseline testing and retesting at year two in reading and spelling, and a nonsignificant decline in mathematic abilities.

This prospective study is still underway and the three-year results have not been fully analyzed. To date, 17 children with posterior fossa tumors who were treated with whole brain radiation therapy have been followed sequentially, tested at baseline, and retested at least three years after diagnosis. FSIQ had fallen for the group as a whole, from a baseline of 103.7 to 90.9, three to four years post-treatment. FSIQ has ranged between 56 and 131 four years posttreatment, a mean drop of 12 IQ points. Similar declines have been found in both verbal and performance IQ scores; and consistent with earlier findings, age was inversely correlated with FSIQ change over time. Those children who were less than seven years old at the time of diagnosis had an overall decline of 27 IQ points on testing at their three to four years follow-up. However, a fall in IQ score was difficult to document in older children. Testing results showed that the most significant drops occurred in the first two years after treatment. Declines in the ensuing years have not been documented. School performance has partially mimicked the falls in IQ scores. All seven children under seven years of age at diagnosis needed some form of special education three to four years later. Of the 10 children who were in school at the time of diagnosis, 40% required special education, 40% required some supportive services such as extra tutoring, and only 20% attended regular classes without additional help. Four of the children initially entered in the prospective study reached the age where they should have graduated from high school, and all four did so. Two are presently in college and two have full time jobs.

DISCUSSION

The results of these prospective studies shed significant light on some of the issues surrounding intellectual sequela in children with MB [17–19]. It is clear that some, but not all children, are significantly damaged. Younger children are at highest risk and suffer significant and progressive falls in intelligence. An extremely disturbing finding in the study report from CHOP is that those children who were under three years of age had more than 30-point falls in IQ scores within two years of treatment. This occurred despite a reduction of the dose of whole brain radiotherapy to 2,400 cGy. This observation led our institution to attempt to reduce the dose of craniospinal radiation even further. The encouraging results of an ongoing protocol coupling radiation therapy with adjuvant chemotherapy (CCNU, vincristine, and cisplatin) have justified a pilot study of lower-dose cranial irradiation. The three-drug regimen and 1,800-cGy whole brain radiation therapy (with a total dose of 5,000–5,500 cGy to the posterior fossa) are employed in all children less than five years with nonmetastatic MB [5]. Only preliminary results of this study are available. The seven children with MB, at a median age of 2.5 years at the time of diagnosis, have not shown an overall fall in IQ scores.

An alternative approach is to utilize chemotherapy alone for young patients with MB. This type of study is presently underway at multiple institutions, including our own. It is unclear whether radiation can be completely obviated in these young patients. There is controversy over whether patients treated with chemotherapy alone at the time of diagnosis, who are in complete remission after a full course of chemotherapy, require consolidation with craniospinal and local boost radiotherapy. There is no evidence that survival can be prolonged with the addition of radiotherapy to the tumor site alone. In fact, in the only recent study to attempt treatment with local radiotherapy and chemotherapy, a high rate of leptomeningeal dissemination was reported [20]. The results of the prospective study of intellect at CHOP strongly suggest that the use of whole brain radiotherapy in the 2,400–3,600. cGy range will result in a significant fall in overall IQ scores in younger patients, for example, three-year-olds.

It must also be stated that it has yet to be shown that chemotherapy is safe insofar as the intellect of children with MB is concerned. Preliminary results have been reassuring in another tumor type, chiasmatic gliomas, treated with actinomycin and vincristine [21]. Children treated on this protocol, without radiation therapy, have yet to suffer a decline in IQ scores over time because of chemotherapy. Results of the use of actinomycin and vincristine obviously cannot be directly extrapolated to MB trials. The drugs used in most MB trials are potentially more neurotoxic.

Retrospective trials in children with MB strongly suggest that the use of methotrexate-based chemotherapy adds to radiation therapy and increases the severity of neurologic complications. In recent studies, the use of intrathecal methotrexate as presymptomatic therapy has been associated with less cognitive damage than whole brain radiation therapy. Our results in three patients with MB, treated only with chemotherapy, have likewise shown no deterioration over time, albeit none of the three received methotrexate. They were treated with CCNU and vincristine, with or without cisplatin. Intellectual sequelae may be seen, however, as chemo-

therapeutic protocols become more aggressive and utilize drugs such as methotrexate or higher doses of chemotherapy that historically have not caused brain injury.

The impact of local radiotherapy on the intellectual sequelae in children treated for MB is impossible to determine from the evidence available. There is no question that parts of the cerebrum are included in the local radiotherapy portal. Portions of the temporal lobes, areas crucial in memory and learning, are included in the radiotherapy ports. The only way to separate the effects of whole brain from local radiotherapy is to study a population of children with tumors that require local radiotherapy alone. Overall survival has been so poor in patients with these types of tumors—primarily brainstem gliomas and ependymomas—that it is practically impossible for any single institution to perform the relevant research. Multiinstitutional studies are needed to evaluate the relationships between local posterior-fossa irradiation and intellectual damage.

Another issue which has yet to be answered by the prospective studies is the impact of whole brain radiotherapy in older children with MB. The results to date suggest that they are less likely to develop severe damage, as measured by drops in overall IQ scores. Nonetheless, clinical impressions and results of school performance evaluations suggest that these children are also impaired by radiotherapy. Defects in memory and in selective aspects of learning are frequent. Stable IQ scores over time in these older patients thus should not be accepted as evidence that radiation therapy is not harmful in adolescents and young adults with MB, but separating the effects of radiotherapy from the impact of other variables has been difficult in this population as it is in others.

Lowering the dose of radiotherapy for children with MB is a two-edged sword.

There are no well-performed dose-response studies determining how much radiation therapy is needed to prevent leptomeningeal relapse in children with MB. There also is no compelling evidence that chemotherapy can effectively reduce the amount of radiotherapy needed. Furthermore, a "safe" dose of radiotherapy, as regards cognitive sequelae, is not known for these children and there are probably inherent factors that make some patients more susceptible to radiation injury than others. A complete delineation of factors associated with declines in intelligence over time and their severity require the completion of well-controlled prospective studies. These entail the evaluation of patients prior to radiation therapy, immediately thereafter, and at fixed follow-up intervals. Given the improving survival rates for children with MB, it is mandatory that any new clinical trial includes prospective neurocognitive assessments as an integral part of the study. This neurocognitive assessment should not be limited only to global assessments of intelligence, but also should include specific measures of neurocognitive function, school performance, and psychosocial development. We thus may have come full circle and must now reassess global scales of function, rather than rely on IQ tests alone.

ACKNOWLEDGMENTS

The author acknowledges the generous support of McDonald Charities.

REFERENCES

1. Allen JC, Bloom J, Ertel I, et al.: Brain tumors in children: Current cooperative and institutional chemotherapy trials in newly diagnosed and recurrent disease. Semin Oncol 13:110–122, 1985.
2. Farwell JR, Dohrmann GJ, Flannery JT: Medulloblastoma in childhood: An epidemiological study. J Neurosurg 61:657–664, 1984.
3. Packer RJ, Siegel KR, Sutton LN, et al.: Efficacy of adjuvant chemotherapy for patients with poor-risk medulloblastoma: A preliminary report. Ann Neurol 24:503–508, 1988.
4. Allen JC, Epstein F: Medulloblastoma and other primary malignant neuroectodermal tumors of the CNS. The effect of patients' age and extent of disease on prognosis. J Neurosurg 57:446–451, 1982.
5. Packer RJ, Sutton LN and D; 'Angio G, et al.: Management of children with primitive neuroectodermal tumors of the posterior fossa/medulloblastoma. Pediatr Neurosci 12:272–282, 1985–1986.
6. Bloom HJC, Wallace ENJ, Henk JM: The treatment and prognosis of medulloblastoma in children: A study of 82 verified cases. Am J Roentgenol 105:43–62, 1969.
7. Jenkin RDT: Medulloblastoma in childhood: Radiation therapy. Canad Med Assoc J 100:51–53, 1969.
8. Bouchard J: Radiation therapy of tumors and disease of the nervous system. Philadelphia: Lea and Febiger, 1966.
9. Raimondi AJ, Tomita T: Medulloblastoma in childhood: Comparative results of partial and total resection. Child Brain 5:310–328, 1979.
10. Spunberg JJ, Chang CH, Goldman M, et al.: Quality of long term survival following irradiation for intracranial tumors in children under the age of two. Int J Radiat Oncol Biol Phys 7:737–736, 1981.
11. Hirsch JF, Renier D, Czernichow P, et al.: Medulloblastoma in childhood. Survival and functional results. Acta Neurochir 48:1–15, 1979.
12. Duffner PK, Cohen ME, Thomas P: Late effects of treatment on the intelligence of children with posterior fossa tumors. Cancer 51:233–237, 1983.
13. Packer RJ, Sposto R, Atkins TE: Quality of life in children with primitive neuroectodermal tumor (medulloblastoma) of the posterior fossa. Pediatr Neurosci 13:169–175, 1988.
14. Danooff BF, Cowchock FS, Marquette C, et al.: Assessment of the long-term effects of primary radiation therapy for brain tumors in children. Cancer 49:1580–1586, 1982.
15. Chin HW, Maruyama Y: Age at treatment and long-term performance results in medulloblastoma. Cancer 53:1952–1958, 1984.
16. Meadows AT, Massari DJ, Fergusson J, et al.: Declines in IQ scores and cognitive dysfunctions in children with acute lymphocytic leukemia treated with cranial irradiation. Lancet 2:1015–1018, 1981.
17. Duffner PK, Cohen ME, Parker MS: Prospective intellectual testing in children with brain tumors. Ann Neurol 23:575–579, 1988.

18. Ellenberg L, McComb JG, Siegel SE, et al.: Factors affecting intellectual outcome in pediatric brain tumor patients. Neurosurgery 21:638–644, 1987.

19. Packer RJ, Sutton LN, Atkins TE, et al.: A prospective study of cognitive function in children receiving whole brain radiotherapy and chemotherapy: 2-year results. J Neurosurg 70:707–713, 1989.

20. Brunat Mentigny M, Bernard JL, Tron P, et al.: Treatment of medulloblastomas with surgery, chemotherapy and radiation therapy limited to the post-fossa and spinal cord. Proceedings of International Society of Pediatric Oncology (SIOP) 58:1986.

21. Packer RJ, Sutton LN, Bilanuik LT et al.: Treatment of chiasmatic hypothalamic gliomas of childhood with chemotherapy. An Update. Ann Neurol 23:79–85, 1988.

7

Physiology of Growth Hormone Production and Release

Charles A. Sklar, M.D.

Growth hormone (GH) is secreted by the anterior pituitary gland and is under the influence of a complex regulatory system that includes both stimulatory and inhibitory factors. Circulating GH appears to exert many of its biologic effects by stimulating the production of insulin-like growth factor-1 (IGF-1) (also known as somatomedin-C) in the liver and other tissues. Circulating IGF-1, in turn, feeds back at the level of the hypothalamus and pituitary to inhibit the secretion of GH. Recent data suggest that it is the IGF-1 produced locally within various tissues, rather than the IGF-1 in the peripheral circulation, that is of primary physiologic importance.

PROCESSING OF GH

Growth hormone is a single-chain polypeptide that contains 191 amino acids. It belongs to a family of polypeptide hormones that includes the placental hormone chorionic somatomammotropin (placental lactogen) and the pituitary hormone prolactin. It is secreted by cells in the anterior pituitary gland known as somatotropes. The human GH genes and the genes for the closely related hormone chorionic somatomammotropin are located in a 50-kB portion of chromosome 17 [1,2]. Five loci reside within the GH gene cluster, including two GH genes. One locus (GH1) encodes for the known protein sequence and is expressed by pituitary tissue. The second locus (GH2) encodes a protein that differs by 13 amino acids and is expressed by the placenta [3].

The major protein formed from the expression of the GH1 gene is a 22-k.dalton GH. It represents the dominant form of GH found in the pituitary gland and the peripheral circulation. Alternative splicing of the GH1 transcript leads to the formation of a 20-k.dalton GH variant that comprises approximately 10% of the total GH within the pituitary gland [4]. Deletion of the GH1 gene is the underlying defect in the rare, familial form of severe isolated GH deficiency known as type 1A [5].

NEUROREGULATION OF GH SECRETION

Growth hormone is secreted episodically in humans. This secretory pattern is felt to result from the interplay between the two hypothalamic neuropeptides, growth hormone–releasing hormone (GHRH) and somatostatin. GHRH stimulates GH production and release, whereas somatostatin exerts an inhibitory effect. Current data support the theory that while GHRH and somatostatin are the primary regulators of GH secretion, a variety of central and peripheral factors are able to modulate GH release by altering the activity of GHRH and/or somatostatin. Many neurotransmitters, including both amine (catecholamine, serotonin, acetylcholine, and histamine) and amino acid

Late Effects of Treatment for Childhood Cancer, pages 49–54 © 1992 Wiley-Liss, Inc.

(β-hydroxybutaric acid) neurotransmitters have the ability to influence GH release [6]. The catecholamine system has been particularly well studied and it is now well established that the α_2-adrenergic system stimulates GH release most probably by augmenting GHRH release. Although only recently appreciated, it is now clear that the cholingergic neuronal system plays an important role in the control of GH release. Muscarinic cholinergic agonists appear to exert their effects by inhibiting somatostatin release [7].

The episodic secretion of GH would appear to result from the episodic secretion of GHRH and somatostatin into the portal circulation, directly influencing anterior pituitary somatotropes. Animal data suggest that these two neuropeptides are released 180 degrees out of phase [8]. A pulse of GH secretion occurs if GHRH is released at a time when somatostatin levels are low. Such reciprocal changes between these neurohormones may be responsible for the ultradian pattern of GH release observed in the peripheral blood.

DYNAMICS OF GH SECRETION

Growth hormone is secreted in episodic bursts throughout the day and night [9]. In humans, GH secretory episodes take place approximately every four hr. The predominant secretory burst of the 24-hr day occurs during the first two hr of nocturnal sleep, coincident with the first episode of slow-wave sleep [10]. The secretory pattern of GH can be affected by a multitude of factors including age, gender, pubertal status, body weight, and nutritional status.

In normal prepubertal children, the integrated concentrations of GH and the 24-hr secretory profiles remain relatively stable [11]. Prior to the onset of puberty, there does not appear to be a correlation with age or gender. A marked increase in GH secretion has been noted in mid-late puberty [11,12]. These increased levels of GH noted at puberty reflect changes in the height or amplitude of the GH pulses and are relatively independent of changes in pulse frequency [12]. The changes in GH secretory dynamics that occur during puberty are mediated, in large part, by the increasing levels of gonadal sex steroids. In children with hypogonadism, the pubertal-rise in GH concentration fails to take place [13]. In late puberty and early adulthood, GH levels return to or below the levels noted in prepubertal children [12]. There is a progressive decline in GH secretion after age 30 years. Important age and sex differences are apparent in adulthood: women produce more GH than men, and older women and men secrete less GH than young women [14]. In adults and the aged of both sexes, there is a strong and direct correlation between GH concentrations and the circulating levels of estradiol [14].

Nutritional status influences GH secretory dynamics. In general, there is an inverse relationship between a person's weight for height (body mass index) and the amount of GH secreted. Obese subjects exhibit blunted GH responses to provocative stimuli that return to normal following appropriate weight reduction [15]. In contrast, both chronic malnutrition and short-term fasting are associated with elevated resting levels of GH [16,17]. A recent study showed that following a 36-hr fast by normal young men, there was a threefold rise in the total GH output because of an augmentation in the amplitude and frequency of GH pulses over 24 hr [17]. The nutrition-related changes in GH secretion are associated with reciprocal variations in the circulating levels of IGF-1.

It is clear that GH is essential for normal linear growth during childhood, but the relationship between GH secretion (amount and pattern), growth rate, and absolute height remains controversial. In broad terms, it seems justified to claim that there is a correlation between growth rate and the amount of GH secreted, since GH deficient children grow slowly and children with GH producing tumors grow at accelerated rates. Whether "short" normal children secrete less GH than "tall" normal children, however, is unresolved. Both Hindmarsh et al. [18] and Albertsson-Wikland and Rosberg [11] found a significant relationship between stature and GH secretion in prepubertal children of varied heights. Hindmarsh et al. [18] further noted that spontaneous GH secretion could best be described in terms of GH pulse amplitude. These data need to be interpreted with caution, however, since in both studies the majority of subjects evaluated had heights outside $=2$ SD of the mean. Studies of spontaneous GH secretion in children of normal stature have consistently revealed that GH concentrations vary widely, with the values in the normal children overlapping those seen in individuals with GH deficiency [19–21]. Moreover, little or no correlation between 24-hr GH concentrations and height has been found in these normally growing children.

GH ACTION

Growth hormone in the peripheral circulation has been shown to exist in a free unbound state and in a bound form complexed to one of a variety of proteins. The major GH binding protein appears to be identical to the extracellular domain of the GH receptor [22]. The physiologic importance of the GH binding protein is not fully understood. Patients with GH resistance resulting from an absence of the GH receptor (Laron-type dwarfism) also lack the GH binding protein [23].

Growth hormone promotes a variety of activities that can be arbitrarily divided into two groups; those that are growth-promoting and insulin-like and those that oppose the action of insulin. The latter activities would appear to be direct effects of GH and include lipolysis, effects on carbohydrate metabolism, and the induction of a vriety of liver enzymes [24]. The growth promoting effects of GH have been considered indirect actions that require the formation of intermediary substances known as somatomedins. The major GH-dependent somatomedin is known as IGF-1 [25]. IGF-1 is a 70 amino acid single-chain polypeptide with considerable homology to the proinsulin molecule. IGF-1 circulates bound in plasma, and the major IGF-1 binding protein is a large molecular weight complex (150K) under GH regulation [26,27]. Circulating levels of IGF-1 are known to be modulated by a variety of factors, including the GH status of the individual, age, nutritional state, and sex steroid milieu.

The conventional and widely held theory (the "somatomedin hypothesis") concerning the growth-promoting actions of GH contends that circulating GH stimulates the liver (and other tissues) to produce IGF-1, which in turn circulates and acts on the growth plate and other target tissue [25]. This is almost certainly an overly simplistic construct. Recent studies from a variety of laboratories indicate that GH and IGF-1 can act in tandem and locally to promote cell proliferation and protein synthesis in both skeletal and nonskeletal tissue. This so-called "dual effector theory" was originally proposed by Green et al. [28]. According to this model, GH stimulates precursor cells to undergo differentiation and IGF-1 acts as a mitogen to promote cell multiplication in young differentiated clones. Studies by Isaksson et al. [29] suggest that GH effects longitudinal bone growth directly by stimulating the differentiation of prechondrocytes in the growth plate. As these cells undergo differentiation, they develop responsiveness to IGF-1 and concomitantly these cells begin to produce IGF-1 locally.

ASSESSMENT OF GH SECRETION

Assessment of GH reserve in the clinical setting has proven to be a difficult and complex task. Because of the pulsatile nature of GH release, random baseline determinations of GH are frequently low and do not allow separation of normals from those with GH deficiency. Despite intensive research, a simple and reliable test for GH reserve has yet to be established. There is a major impediment to achieving this goal. Criteria for normality are lacking and the parameters of GH release (e.g., total amount produced, number of pulses, and height of the pulses) critical for normal growth remain unclear.

For the past several decades, a variety of provocative agents capable of stimulating GH release have been utilized to assess GH reserve [30]. Included among these are insulin-hypoglycemia, intravenous arginine HCl, oral L-DOPA, and oral Clonidine. These pharmacologic stimulation tests appear to have a high level of diagnostic accuracy. Growth hormone responses following these agents correlate well with physiologic tests of GH secretion [31,32] (e.g., 24-hr integrated concentrations of GH and peak GH level during sleep). Nonetheless, a number of unresolved problems exist with current provocative tests. First, control data for children of different ages and varying pubertal status have never been developed. Second, discordant results can be obtained with different agents, and it is unclear what if any clinical significance this may have. Third, different GH immunoassay systems give discrepant potency estimates that complicate interpretation of the test results [33,34]. Finally, several recent reports suggest that certain individuals with normal reponses to pharmacologic tests may have subnormal endogenous GH secretion over 24 hr [35,36]. This discrepancy between the results of pharmacologic and physiologic GH tests

seems to be particularly common among subjects previously treated with cranial irradiation [37]. Some have suggested, therfore, that measurement of spontaneous GH over 12–24 hr would be highly sensitive and offer clear advantages over pharmacologic tests. The work of Rose et al. [19], however, failed to demonstrate any diagnostic advantage of the measurement of spontaneous secretion of GH over routine provocative tests in a group of prepubertal short children.

Measurement of the IGF-1 concentration in plasma must be viewed as a screening procedure and does not provide a substitute for more direct assessments of GH secretion. Although children with classic GH deficiency generally have IGF-1 levels below age adjusted norms, very young children and short-normals of any age will often have IGF-1 values that overlap those seen in true GH deficiency [38,39]. Furthermore, chronically ill children and individuals with borderline nutrition may have low IGF-1 levels despite normal GH status. The GH response to synthetic GHRH has proven, likewise, to have limited clinical utility owing to the wide range of responses observed in both normal subjects and those with GH deficiency [40].

The measurement of urinary GH and the determination of the plasma concentration of the GH-dependent IGF-1 binding protein have recently been utilized to assess endogenous GH secretion [41,42]. Both these techniques are relatively simple and inexpensive and they appear to correlate well with the individual's GH status. Additional data are required, however, before either technique can be recommended for routine clinical use.

REFERENCES

1. Phillips JA III, Parks JS, Hjelle BL, et al.: Genetic basis of familial growth hormone deficiency type 1. J Clin Invest 70:489–495, 1982.
2. Hirt H, Kimelman J, Birnbaum MJ, et al.: The

human growth hormone gene locus: structure, evolution, and allelic variations. DNA 6:59–70, 1987.

3. Seebergh PH: The human growth hormone gene family: nucleotide sequeces show recent divergence and predict a new polypeptide hormone. DNA 1:239–249, 1982.

4. Lewis VJ: Variants of growth hormone and prolactin and their post-translational modifications. Annu Rev Physiol 46:33–42, 1984.

5. Phillips JA III, Hjelle BL, Seeburg PH, et al.: Molecular basis for familial isolated growth hormone deficiency. Proc Natl Acad Sci USA 78:6372–6375, 1981.

6. Muller EE, Locatelli V, Cella SG, et al.: The role of neurotransmitters in growth hormone secretion. In Bercu, BB (ed): Basic and Clinical Aspects of Growth Hormone. New York: Plenum, 1988, pp 83–94.

7. Richardson SB, Hollander CS, D'Elatto D, et al.: Acetylcholine inhibits the release of somatostatin from rat hypothalamus in vitro. Endocrinology 107:1837–1842, 1980.

8. Tannenbaum GS and Ling N: The interrelationship of growth hormone (GH)-releasing factor and somatostatin in generation of the ultradian rhythm of GH secretion. Endocrinology 115:1952–1957, 1984.

9. Quabbe H-J, Schilling E, Helge H: Pattern of growth hormone secretion during a 24-hour fast in normal adults. J Clin Endocrinol Metab 26: 173–177, 1966.

10. Takaahashi Y, Kipnis DM, Daughaday WH: Growth hormone secretion during sleep. J Clin Invest 47:2079–2090, 1968.

11. Albertsson-Wikland K, Rosberg S: Analyses of 24-hour growth hormone profiles in children: relation to growth. J Clin Endocrinol Metab 67: 493–500, 1988.

12. Martha RM Jr, Rogol AD, Veldhuis JD, et al.: Alterations in the pulsatile properties of circulating growth hormone concentrations during puberty in boys. J Clin Endocrinol Metab 69:563–570, 1989.

13. Ross JL, Long LM, Lorieux DL, Cutler GM Jr: Growth hormone secretory dynamices in Turner syndrome. J Pediatr 106:202–206, 1935.

14. Ho KY, Evans WS, Blizzard RM, et al.: Effects of sex and age on the 24-hour profile of growth hormone secretion in man: importance of endogenous estradiol concentrations. J Clin Endocrinol Metab 64:51–58, 1987.

15. Williams T, Berelowitz M, Joffe SN, et al.: Impaired growth hormone responses to growth hormone-releasing factor in obesity. A pituitary defect reversed with weight reduction. N Engl J Med 34:1403–1407, 1984.

16. Soliman AT, Hassan AEHI, Aref MK, et al.: Serum insulin-like growth factors I and II concentrations and growth hormone and insulin responses to arginine infusion in children with protein-energy malnutrition before and after nutritional rehabilitation. Pediatr Res 20:1122–1130, 1986.

17. Ho KY, Veldhuis JD, Johnson ML, et al.: Fasting enhances growth hormone secretion and amplifies the complex rhythms of growth hormone secretion in man. J Clin Invest 81:968–975, 1988.

18. Hindmarsh P, Smith PJ, Brook CGD, Mathews DR: The relationship between height velocity and growth hormone secretion in short prepubertal children. Clin Endocrinol 27:581, 1987.

19. Rose SR, Ross JL, Uriate M, et al.: The advantage of measuring stimulated as compared with spontaneous growth hormone levels in the diagnosis of growth hormone deficiency. N Engl J Med 319:201–207, 1988.

20. Costin G, Kaufman FR, Brasel JA: Growth hormone secretory dynamics in subjects with normal stature. J Pediatr 115:537–544, 1989.

21. Lin T-H, Kirkland RT, Sherman BM, Kirkland JL: Growth hormone testing in short children and their response to growth hormone therapy. J Pediatr 115:57–63, 1989.

22. Baumann G, Shaw MA: Immuno-chemical similarity of the human plasma growth hormone-binding protein and the rabbit liver growth hormone receptor. Biochem Biophys Res Commun 152:573–578, 1988.

23. Baumann G, Shaw MA, Winter RJ: Absence of the plasma growth hormone-binding protein in Laron-type dwarfism. J Clin Endocrinol Metab 65:814–816, 1987.

24. Van Wyk JJ, Casella SJ, Hynes M, Lund PK: Indirect actions of growth hormone. In Underwood LE (ed): Human Growth Hormone. Progress and Challenges. New York: Marcel Dekker, 1988, pp 25–61.

25. Van Wyk JJ, Underwood LE, Hintz RL, et al.: The somatomedins: A family of insulin-like hormones under growth hormone control. Rec Prog Horm Res 30:259–318, 1974.

26. Hintz RL, Liu F: Demonstration of specific plasma protein binding sites for somatomedin. J Clin Endocrinol Metab 45:989–995, 1977.

27. Cohen KL, Nissley SP: The serum half-life of somatomedin activity: evidence for growth hormone dependence. Acta Endocrinologica 83:243–258, 1976.

28. Green H, Morikawa M, Nixon T: A dual effector theory of growth-hormone action. Differentation 29:195–198, 1985.

29. Isaksson OGP, Lindhahl A, Nilsson A and

Isgaard J: Mechanism of stimulatory effect of growth hormone on longitudinal bone growth. Endocrinol Rev 8:426–438, 1987.

30. Frasier SD: A review of growth hormone stimulation tests in children. Pediatrics 53:929–937, 1974.

31. Plotnick LP, Lee PA, Migeon CJ, Kowarski AA: Comparison of physiological and pharmacological tests of growth hormone function in children with short stature. J Clin Endocrinol Metab 48:811–815, 1979.

32. Hindmarsh PC, Smith PJ, Taylor BJ, et al.: Comparison between a physiological and a pharmacological stimulus of growth hormone secretion: response to stage IV sleep and insulin-induced hypoglycemia. Lancet 2:1033–1035, 1985.

33. Reiter EO, Morris AH, MacGillivray MH, Weber D: Variable estimates of serum growth hormone concentrations by different radioassay systems. J Clin Endocrinol Metab 66:68–71, 1988.

34. Celniker AC, Chen AB, Wert RM Jr, Sherman BM: Variability in the quantitation of circulating growth hormone using commercial immunoassays. J Clin Endocrinol Metab 68:469–476, 1989.

35. Spiliotis BE, August GP, Hung W, et al.: Growth hormone neurosecretory dysfunction: a treatable cause of short stature. JAMA 251:2223–2230, 1984.

36. Bercu BB, Shulman D, Root AW, Spiolitis BE: Growth hormone (GH) provocative testing frequently does not reflect endogenous GH secretion. J Clin Endocrinol Metab 63:709–716, 1986.

37. Blatt J, Bercu BB, Gillin JC, et al.: Reduced pulsatile growth hormone secretion in children after therapy for acute leukemia. J Pediatr 108:182–186, 1984.

38. Underwood LE, D'Ercole AJ, Van Wyk JJ: Somatomedin-C and the assessment of growth. Pediatr Clin North Am 27:771–782, 1980.

39. Rosenfeld RG, Wilson DM, Lee PDK, Hintz RL: Insulin-like growth factors I and II in evaluation of growth retardation. J Pediatr 109:428–433, 1986.

40. Chalew SA, Armour KM, Levin PA, et al.: Growth hormone (GH) response to GH-releasing hormone in children with subnormal integrated concentrations of GH. J Clin Endocrinol Metab 62:1110–1115, 1986.

41. Albini CH, Quattrin T, Vandlen RL, MacGillivray MH: Quantitation of urinary growth hormone in children with normal and abnormal growth. Pediatr Res 23:89–92, 1988.

42. Blum WF, Ranke MB, Kietzmann K, et al.: A specific radioimmunoassay for the growth hormone ((GH)-dependent somatomedin-binding protein: its use for diagnosis of GH deficiency. J Clin Endocrinol Metab 70:1292–1298, 1990.

8

Thyroid and Gonadal Function and Growth of Long-Term Survivors of Medulloblastoma/PNET

Sharon E. Oberfield, M.D., Charles Sklar, M.D., Jeffrey Allen, M.D., Russell Walker, M.D., Mary McElwain, M.S.N, Vassilios Papadakis, M.D., Janine Maenza, M.D., Steven Ralston, M.D., and Lenore S. Levine, M.D.

Medulloblastoma (MB) or primitive neuroectodermal tumors (PNET) comprise 15–20% of all primary brain tumors in childhood [1]. Treatment with surgery followed by craniospinal radiation with or without additional adjuvant chemotherapy has resulted in a 50–60% five-year survival [2,3]. It is now well established that unfortunate major endocrinologic sequelae occur in long-term survivors of MB/PNET [4]. The most obvious disturbance is that of growth retardation [5–6]. Abnormal growth appears to be related to the age at irradiation, dosage of spinal irradiation, chemotherapy regimen, as well as the presence of concomitant thyroid and gonadal dysfunction [7–10]. We report here endocrine function in patients with MB followed since 1979 and height data in 14 who have completed their growth.

METHODS

Study Population

The study was designed to continue long-term surveillance of 22 patients with MB/PNET initially reported in 1986 [11], as well as to evaluate new patients for ongoing prospective assessment of endocrine function. Thirty-six patients (22 males) were studied. Their ages were $2\frac{1}{2}$–$23^{8}/_{12}$ years (mean: 9.4 years) at time of diagnosis. The patients are currently $1^{5}/_{12}$–$14^{7}/_{12}$ years postdiagnosis and were studied as early as four months after diagnosis. All patients received at least 2,400 cGy to the craniospinal axis and at least 5,000 cGy (total) to the posterior fossa as previously described [11]. Eighteen patients received chemotherapy which, in the majority, included CCNU, vincristine, and prednisone (CCSG 942). The remainder were enrolled on CCSG 921 Regimen A (3 drugs) or Regimen B (8 drugs). The mean dose of radiation was equivalent in those who received radiotherapy (RT) as compared to those who received RT and chemotherapy. Six had died, all from recurrence of the primary tumor.

The investigations were approved by the Institutional Review Boards of the New York Hospital Cornell University Medical Center, Memorial Sloan-Kettering Cancer Center, and New York University Medical Center. Informed consent had been obtained from all patients. Repeat studies were performed as part of standard patient care.

Pubertal status was defined according to the stages of Tanner [13]. Testicular size was measured with the Prader orchido-

Late Effects of Treatment for Childhood Cancer, pages 55–62 © 1992 Wiley-Liss, Inc.

meter. Bone age was evaluated according to the standards of Greulich and Pyle [14]. Upper/lower segment ratios were measured by determining total height and pubis to floor length. Final height was defined as a growth rate of less than 1.2 cm over the previous year in fully pubertal or post menarchal patients [15].

Hormonal Evaluation

Thyrotropin releasing hormone, 7 µg/kg, was given by rapid intravenous infusion. Stimulation tests for evaluation of growth hormone (GH) included: exercise test (20 min), glucagon (0.1 mg/kg IM, maximum dose 1 mg); insulin-induced hypoglycemia (0.1 U/kg); L-DOPA (250 mg PO for body weight <30 kg or 500 mg PO for ≥30 kg), clonidine (150 µg/m²); and arginine (0.5 g/kg IV; maximum 30 g). Any patient who was not euthyroid at the time of the initial GH evaluation underwent repeat evaluation in the euthyroid state. Growth hormone deficiency was defined as a peak GH level < 7 ng/ml in response to pharmacologic testing. Growth hormone therapy was administered in doses of 0.05–0.1 mg/kg three times a week by IM or SQ injections. Growth hormone, T4, T3, TSH, LH, and FSH were measured by modifications of standard radioimmunoassays.

Statistical Analysis

Statistical comparisons were made using the Student's *t*-test, and the chi-square test of homogeneity of proportions. Life tables were constructed using standard methods [16,17].

RESULTS

Growth

Thirty-two of 36 patients had not yet completed their final growth prior to the time of diagnosis. Twenty-four of these 32 patients had abnormal growth rates (Figs.

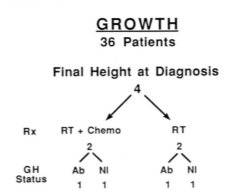

Fig. 1. Treatment and growth status in four patients who had achieved final height prior to diagnosis.

1 and 2). The abnormal growth rates were noted in 3/3 diagnosed prior to age 3, 17/23 at ages 3–10, and 4/6 more than 10 years of age. Bone ages were within one year of chronologic age at the time of initial testing in 21 patients, delayed in six, and accelerated in two. Twenty-one of 24 patients with abnormal growth rates underwent GH testing; 14 were deficient (8/14 who received RT and chemotherapy and 6/10 who received RT alone). Among the eight patients with normal growth rates, three of the seven tested

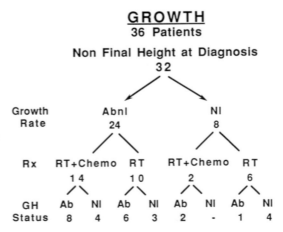

Fig. 2. Treatment and growth status in 32 patients who had not achieved final height prior to diagnosis.

were noted to be GH-deficient (2/2 who received RT and chemotherapy and 1/6 who received RT alone). Thus, 17 of the 28 patients (61%) who had not achieved final height at the time of initial diagnosis and who underwent GH stimulation testing were GH-deficient.

An abnormal response to GH testing was observed as early as six months to as late as three years after completion of therapy.

Twelve patients (8 GH-deficient) have been treated with GH. The mean growth rate during the first year of treatment (N = 12) was 6.3 cm (3.7 − 10 cm). During the second year of treatment (N = 7) the mean rate was 4.27 cm (2.1 − 5.8 cm) and in the third year of treatment the mean growth rate was 4.3 cm (1.9 − 8.2 cm). One patient continued to receive GH for a fourth year and grew at a negligible rate of 1.5 cm/year.

Fourteen patients at the time of this report have achieved final heights (Tables 1 and 2, Figs. 3 and 4). Six of these patients (4 GH-deficient) were treated with GH and have reached a final height less than the fifth percentile, standard deviation score (SDS) − 5.3 to −2.5. Eight other patients were not treated with GH; five

reached final heights greater than the fifth percentile; SDS −0.15 to −0.1. None of these children was GH-deficient. The other three patients not treated with GH (2 GH-deficient and 1 not tested) had a final height under the fifth percentile, SDS −5 to −2.4. The mean age of diagnosis (11.5 years) of the children who achieved final height greater than the fifth percentile (N = 5) was significantly greater than the mean age at diagnosis (6.45 years) of the children whose final height was less than the fifth percentile (N = 9, $P < 0.005$). An additional interesting fact is that 5/7 of the patients who had completed their growth and who received RT alone had a final height that was greater than the fifth percentile, whereas none of the seven who received RT and chemotherapy had a final height greater than the fifth percentile. Of the 14 patients who had achieved final height, upper/lower segment ratios were measured in seven and ranged from 0.78–0.93.

THYROID ASSESSMENT

Abnormal thyroid function was observed in 21/36 patients, consistent with primary hypothyroidism in 19 and with

TABLE 1. Clinical Data in Patients Achieving Final Height Less Than 5th Percentile

Patient no.	Sex	Age at Dx (years)	Rx	GH status	SDS score
			GH Rx (6)		
2	M	7 $^{11}/_{12}$	RT+Chemo	Ab	−5.3
3	M	6 $^{7}/_{12}$	RT+Chemo	Ab	−2.5
7	M	6 $^{11}/_{12}$	RT+Chemo	NI	−2.9
11	F	7 $^{6}/_{12}$	RT+Chemo	Ab	−4.2
14	F	5 $^{4}/_{12}$	RT	NI	−3.1
25	F	3 $^{4}/_{12}$	RT+Chemo	Ab	−4.1
			NonGH Rx (3)		
1	F	4 $^{4}/_{12}$	RT+Chemo	Ab	−3.0
10	F	2 $^{6}/_{12}$	RT+Chemo	not tested	−5.0
15	M	12 $^{1}/_{12}$	RT	Ab	−2.4

TABLE 2. Clinical Data in Patients Achieving Final Height Greater Than 5th Percentile[a]

Patient no.	Sex	Age at Dx (years)	Rx	GH status	SDS score
4	M	13 4/12	RT	NI	−0.1
13	M	12 11/12	RT	NI	−1.1
17	M	9 9/12	RT	NI	−1.5
19	M	12 4/12	RT	NI	−0.8
9	F	9	RT	NI	−0.5

[a] None treated with GH.

hypothalamic hypothyroidism in two. Among the 21 patients, 13 of 18 treated with both RT and chemotherapy and 8 of 18 treated with RT alone developed abnormal thyroid function. It was first observed six months to 6½ years after therapy. Life table analysis curves predicted that 100% of the patients who received both RT and chemotherapy would have primary hypothyroidism by 90 months postdiagnosis. By contrast, only 50% of patients who received RT alone had abnormal thyroid function 120 months postdiagnosis (Fig. 5). These results approached but did not reach statistical significance by chi-square test for homogeneity of proportions ($P = 0.087$). Fourteen of 19 patients who had not finished growing at the time of initial assessment had both abnormal thyroid function on initial testing and abnormal growth rates.

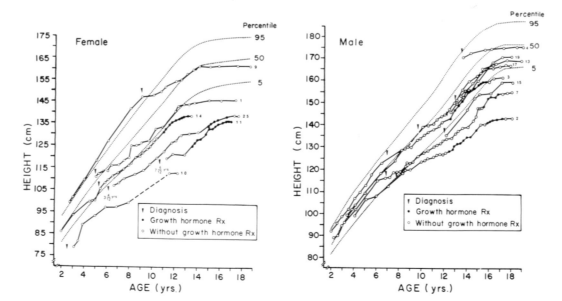

Fig. 3. Growth curves for female patients who have achieved final heights.

Fig. 4. Growth curves for male patients who have achieved final heights.

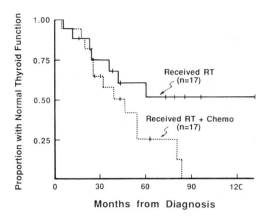

Fig. 5. Time to thyroid dysfunction (primary hypothyroidism) in patients receiving radiation or radiation and chemotherapy for MB/PNET.

PUBERTAL ASSESSMENT

Abnormal pubertal progression was observed in 13 patients (Table 3). Six, including two males, had primary gonadal failure judged by elevated gonadotropin levels. Nine of 13 received both chemotherapy and RT. Because many of the total patient population have not yet completed puberty, it is probable that additional disturbances will be observed.

DISCUSSION

The current study further demonstrated the high incidence of disordered growth, as well as thyroid and gonadal dysfunction, in children who received cranio-spinal radiotherapy and chemotherapy for MB. Since our original prospective study [11], reports of therapy-associated complications have increased. However, few have addressed the issue of the final height attained by children with or without GH therapy [18]. Clayton et al. [19] did not find a significant difference in the growth response to GH therapy in seven children who had received cranial irradiation as compared to GH-treated patients with idiopathic GH deficiency. In the cranial irradiation group, however, they demonstrated that the mean bone age at the onset of puberty was younger although the duration of puberty was normal. Therefore, despite a normal duration of puberty, the children had less actual time available for growth hormone treatment and completed their growth earlier. Only three of their seven patients reached a final height >3% [19]. Clayton et al. [20] also reported 19 patients who had received craniospinal irradiation and were treated with GH. Eight completed final growth. A significant improvement in leg length on GH treatment was observed, but the patients still lost 0.9 SD of standing height. This was better, however, than the 1.7 SD loss seen in similarly treated patients who did not receive GH. Ahmed et al. [21] also studied the growth patterns of children who received both cranial and spinal irradiation. Final height obtained in three patients with MB was similar to that

TABLE 3. Pubertal Dysfunction in 13 Patients

	RT and chemotherapy		RT alone	
	No.	Age at Dx	No.	Age at Dx
Delayed puberty	2	3 $^{11}/_{12}$, 10 $^{1}/_{12}$[a]	—	
Early puberty	1	6 $^{10}/_{12}$[a]	—	
Irregular menses	1	4 $^{11}/_{12}$	2	5 $^{4}/_{12}$, 23 $^{8}/_{12}$
↑ Gonadotropins	4	6 $^{5}/_{12}$, 12 $^{1}/_{12}$, 7 $^{6}/_{12}$, 9 $^{8}/_{12}$[a]	2	4 $^{11}/_{12}$, 3 $^{1}/_{12}$[a]
Firm testes	1	7 $^{11}/_{12}$[a]		

[a] Male

of our patients (SDS -2.6 to -3.7) despite treatment with GH. Lannering and Albertsson-Wikland [22] assessed 15 patients who received cranial irradiation including seven with MB/PNET or ependymoma. Four of the seven received spinal irradiation. With GH treatment, catch-up growth was observed over a one-year period. They demonstrated that those given craniospinal irradiation grew below the mean growth rate increment observed for the total group during their GH treatment. That study, however, did not include final height data [22]. Recently, Rappaport and Brauner [10] documented a final height loss of 1.4 SD in patients who had been treated for MB. The loss could be attributed in part to lack of spinal growth and was most significant in children who were under six years of age when irradiated. In our study, as shown in Tables 1 and 2 and Figures 3 and 4, 9 of 14 patients achieved a final height that was significantly below their pretreatment height potential. Despite the reasonable first year response to GH, many patients had less than optimal responses in subsequent years, as has been reported by others [5]. In addition, although puberty was not precocious in our population, it came relatively early and resulted in a rapid decrease in growth potential. Our patients' data suggest that growth impairment was observed equally in patients who received RT or RT and chemotherapy; but none of those patients whose final height was greater than the fifth percentile had received chemotherapy. It is possible that this finding occurs because these patients were older at time of diagnosis. This is in agreement with the data of Brauner et al. [9], who suggested that children who were younger at diagnosis fared less well. Of most concern is that treatment with GH did not appear to significantly change the final height of our patients who were growing abnormally. Since many of them received GH therapy

at a late age, timing may well be the important factor. Furthermore, lack of attainment of adequate final height results in part from truncal shortening secondary to RT as previously reported [23].

Most of our patients had evidence of primary hypothyroidism. This is not unanticipated since the mean calculated radiation dose to the thyroid was close to 2,400 cGy [11]. Livesey and Brook [24] recently reported that 69% of their population who had spinal irradiation and chemotherapy had elevated thyroid stimulating hormone (TSH) levels and that chemotherapy appeared to be additive with respect to thyroid dysfunction. We also observed a greater chance of having abnormal thyroid function if the treatment regimen included both RT and chemotherapy. However, this finding did not reach statistical significance in our small number of patients.

Primary gonadal failure is a well-recognized complication of therapy for CNS tumors. Primary gonadal dysfunction can occur following treatment with either chemotherapy (primarily the nitrosoureas BCNU and CCNU) [25–27] and/or spinal irradiation [28]. There are important sex differences, however. Following spinal RT alone, the incidence of ovarian failure is much higher than the incidence of testicular failure [25,28,29]. Ovarian dysfunction after treatment with CCNU is often transient and reversible [27], whereas in the majority of boys, chemotherapy-induced gonadal failure appears to be long-lasting [26]. In the current study, we identified six individuals with primary gonadal failure as judged by raised baseline levels of gonadotropins. Four received both spinal irradiation and chemotherapy; the other two (one male and one female) received only craniospinal irradiation. These data support the contention that scattered radiation from spinal fields can cause damage to the testis as well as to the ovary [28,30]. The implications of these findings vis-a-vis our patients' sexual maturation and future fertility remain unclear.

In summary, although long-term survival has been achieved in a number of children who are now entering adulthood, many of these individuals have major endocrinopathies. Our experience would suggest that after the first year posttreatment, if inadequate growth is observed, patients should be offered therapy with GH. Clinicians should also be aware that earlier onset of puberty may occur in this population and may confound interpretation of the adequacy of growth rates. In addition, all patients should continually be screened for development of thyroid disturbances; we continue to recommend replacement therapy whenever abnormalities are discovered. It is hoped that through collaborative efforts aimed at reducing the radiation dosage delivered to the craniospinal axis and the earlier initiation of GH treatment, each patient's full height potential may be more nearly achieved.

REFERENCES

1. Silverberg E, Lubera JA: Cancer statistics 1988. Cancer 38:5–22, 1988.
2. Allen JC, Bloom J, Ertel I, et al.: Brain tumors in children: Current cooperative and institutional chemotherapy trials in newly diagnosed recurrent disease. Semin Oncol 13:110–122, 1985.
3. Packer RJ, Sutton LN, D'Angio G, Evans AE, Shut L: Management of children with primitive neuroectodermal tumors of the posterior fossa/medulloblastoma. Pediatr Neurosci 12:272–282, 1986.
4. Duffner PK, Cohen ME, Thomas P, Lansky SB: The long term effects of cranial irradiation on the central nervous system. Cancer 56:1841–1847, 1985.
5. Rappaport R, Fontoura M, Brauner R: Growth hormone secretion and growth in central nervous system irradiated children. In International Symposium on Growth Hormone: Basic and Clinical Aspects. Tampa: Plenum, 1988, pp 143–155.
6. Costin G: Effects of low dose cranial radiation on growth hormone secretory dynamics and hypothalamic-pituitary function. Am J Dis Child 142:847–852, 1988.
7. Shalet SM, Clayton PE, Price DA: Growth impairment following treatment for childhood brain tumors. Acta Paediatr Scand (Suppl) 343:137–145, 1988.
8. Albertsson-Wikland K, Lannering B, Marky F, Mellander L, Wannholt U: A longitudinal study on growth and spontaneous growth hormone (GH) secretion in children with irradiated brain tumors. Acta Paediatr Scand 76:966–973, 1987.
9. Brauner R, Rappaport R, Prevot C, Czernichow P, Zucker JM, Bataini P, Lemerle J, Sarrazin D, Guyda HJ: A prospective study of the development of growth hormone deficiency in children given cranial irradiation and its relation to statural growth. J Clin Endocrinol Metab 68: 346–351, 1989.
10. Rappaport R, Brauner R: Growth and endocrine disorders secondary to cranial irradiation. Pediatr Res 25:561–567, 1989.
11. Oberfield SE, Allen JC, Pollack J, New MI, Levine LS: Long-term endocrine sequelae after treatment of medulloblastoma: Prospective study of growth and thyroid function. J Pediatr 108:219–223, 1986.
12. Jereb B, Reid A, Ahuja R: Patterns of failure in patients with medulloblastoma. Cancer 50:2941, 1982.
13. Tanner JM, Whitehouse RW: Longitudinal standards for height, weight, velocity and stages of puberty. Arch Dis Child 51:170, 1976.
14. Greulich WW, Pyle SI (eds): Radiographic Atlas of Skeletal Development of the Hands and Wrist. Stanford, CA: Stanford University Press, 1959.
15. Roche AF: The final phase of growth in stature. Growth, Genetics and Hormones 5:4–6, 1989.
16. Snedecor GW, Cochran WG (eds): Statistical Methods (7th ed). Ames, IA: Iowa State University, 1980, pp 100–105.
17. Peto R, Pike M, Armitage P, Breslow NE, Cox DR, Howard SV, Mantel N, McPherson K, Peto J, Smith PG: Design and analysis of randomized trials requiring prolonged observation of each patient. II. Analysis and examples. Br J Cancer 35:1, 1977.
18. Shalet SM, Clayton PE, Price DA: Growth and pituitary function in children treated for brain tumors or acute lymphoblastic leukemia. Horm Res 30:53–61, 1988.
19. Clayton PE, Shalet SM, Price DA: Growth response to growth hormone therapy following cranial irradiation. Eur J Pediatr 147:593–596, 1988.
20. Clayton PE, Shalet SM, Price DA: Growth response to growth hormone therapy following

craniospinal irradiation. Eur J Pediatr 147:597–601, 1988.

21. Ahmed SR, Shalet SM, Beardwell CG: The effects of cranial irradiation on growth hormone secretion. Acta Paediatr Scand 75:255–260, 1986.

22. Lannering B, Albertsson-Wikland K: Improved growth response to GH treatment in irradiated children. Acta Paediatr Scand 78:562–567, 1989.

23. Probert JC, Parker BR, Kaplan HS: Growth retardation in children after megavoltage irradiation of the spine. Cancer 32:634–639, 1973.

24. Livesey EA, Brook CGD: Thyroid dysfunction after radiotherapy and chemotherapy of brain tumors. Arch Dis Child 64:593–595, 1989.

25. Livesey EA, Brook CGD: Gonadal dysfunction after treatment of intracranial tumors. Arch Dis Child 63:495–500, 1989.

26. Clayton PE, Shalet SM, Price DA, et al.: Testicular damage after chemotherapy for childhood brain tumors. J Pediatr 112:922–926, 1988.

27. Clayton PE, Shalet SM, Price DA: Ovarian function following chemotherapy of childhood brain tumors. Med Pediatr Oncol 17:92–96, 1989.

28. Brown IH, Lee TJ, Eden OB, et al.: Growth and endocrine function after treatment for medulloblastoma. Arch Dis Child 58:722–727, 1983.

29. Ahmed SR, Shalet SM, Campbell RHA, et al.: Primary gonadal damage following treatment of brain tumors. J Pediatr 103:562–565, 1983.

30. Sklar CA, Robison LL, Nesbit ME, et al.: Effects of radiation on testicular function in long-term survivors of childhood acute lymphoblastic leukemia. A Report from the Childrens Cancer Study Group. J Clin Oncol 8:1981–1987, 1990.

9

Effects of Irradiation on Skeletal Growth and Development

Sarah S. Donaldson, M.D.

The inhibitory effects of radiation on growing bone were first described by Perthes in 1903 [1], who noted that a chicken irradiated to one wing demonstrated retarded growth as compared to the nonirradiated wing. Later, Fosterling [2] made a similar observation following hemibody radiation in experimental rabbits. The skeletal effects of radiation and its effect upon bone growth, the development of scoliosis, radiation induced necrosis, and induction of malignancy has stimulated descriptive documentaries and reviews [3].

The major variables relating to these skeletal effects that have been implicated are:

1. Age at the time of treatment.
2. Quality of radiation, dose per fraction, and total dose.
3. Volume irradiated.
4. Growth potential of the treated site.
5. Individual genetic and familial factors.
6. Coexisting therapy—surgery and chemotherapy [4,5].

While many authors have repeatedly depicted the deleterious effects of ionizing radiation, none to date have effectively quantitated the damage, or provided dose/volume/age guidelines with which risk of injury can be compared against efficacy of treatment. Predictive assays to estimate extent of injury have not been validated.

PATHOPHYSIOLOGY

The pathophysiologic changes of radiation injury to bone were traditionally thought to be secondary to vascular fibrosis, but more recently have been considered to be a result of direct intracellular damage of the chondroblasts, leading to arrest and destruction [6–8]. The morphologic changes that appear following radiation to the growing skeleton are known more from studies in animals than in humans. In growing rodents, a single fraction of 600 cGy can cause reduction in mitotic activity in the zone of proliferating chondroblasts [7,8]. Radiation causes an inhibition of proliferation of cartilage cells, a decrease in cellularity and disarray of the cellular columns within a growth plate, and ultimately necrosis. Simultaneously, vascular changes occur. Intermitotic chondroblasts are the most radiosensitive cells of the skeleton. Osteoblasts are much less sensitive, but are damaged with high doses of radiation. Osteoclastic activity is related to the integrity of the bone marrow and blood vessels. Vascular injury leads to impaired reabsorption of bone and cartilage. The effect on bone growth is attributed to the loss of proliferating cells at the growth plate, the decreased ability of surviving cells to synthesize matrix, and/or the production of an abnormal matrix that fails to calcify. Progressively ischemic bone is susceptible to stress, and fractures may occur (Fig. 1). Repair from trauma or

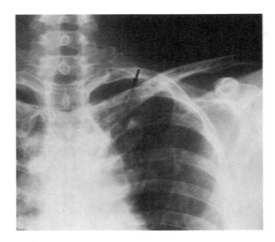

Fig. 1. At age 14, this boy underwent 45.0 Gy to a mantle field for treatment of Hodgkin's disease. Six months after completion of therapy, he suffered a left neck recurrence and received a second course of therapy (45.0 Gy to the left supraclavicular fossa or a total of 90.0 Gy within a one-year period). He remains free of disease. Twenty-three years later, he experienced a left clavicular fracture in the field of high-dose radiation (arrow).

infection is also limited resulting in poor healing of irradiated bone. Evidence of focal muscular atrophy, ischemia, and vascular injury may also appear in skeletal muscle. These changes are not, however, specific to irradiation injury, and morphologically are similar to the myopathic process seen in collagen–vascular disease or in genetic disorders [9].

The epiphysis-physis portion of a long bone appears to be the most sensitive to radiation, which causes an arrest of chondrogenesis resulting in a short bone. Irradiation to the metaphysis results in a failure of the absorptive process of calcified cartilage and bone, resulting in metaphyseal flaring due to selective interruption of bone reabsorption. Diaphyseal irradiation produces errors of modeling with a decrease in periosteal activity leading to long thin bones with a tendency to fracture [10]. There is little alteration in bone growth with total fractionated doses of irradiation less than 10 Gy. Doses of 10–20 Gy produce partial growth arrest, often with transverse bone lines, and doses much greater than 20 Gy are required to completely arrest endochondral bone formation [11].

CLINICAL EXPERIENCE

Prediction of extremity growth in children and the relative contribution from the proximal versus the distal end of long bones (humerus, femur, and tibia) have been investigated. Anderson et al. [12] showed that in a femur, approximately 30% of growth comes from the proximal epipyhysis, while 70% comes from the distal epiphysis. In the tibia, 60% of growth is contributed by the proximal, and 40% comes from the distal end of the bone. In the humerus, however, 80% of growth comes from the proximal epiphysis, while approximately 20% arises from the distal growth center.

The lower femoral epiphysis provides ³⁄₈ of an inch per year, while the upper tibial epiphysis provides ¼ of an inch of growth per year [13,14]. In general, the age of cessation of growth in boys is 16 years, while in girls it is 14 years. Thus, one can estimate the percentage deficit that might result from a course of external beam radiotherapy by knowing the volume and site of an irradiated field, the radiation dose needed for tumor control, and the percentage of growth stemming from the volume of interest. This is particularly true regarding an extremity when a growth plate is included in a radiotherapy field, as leg/length discrepancy by epiphyseal arrest has been thoroughly studied [13].

However, growth disturbance from radiotherapy in the axial skeleton, as opposed to the appendicular skeleton, represents a problem more difficult to quantitate precisely and predict prospectively. Probert and Parker [10] were the first investigators to quantitate bone growth alteration related to megavoltage radiotherapy. They described a disproportionate alteration in sitting height as compared to standing height among a group of children with medulloblastoma, acute lymphocytic leukemia, and Hodgkin's disease who received megavoltage radiation to the entire spine. They divided their patient population into those receiving high-dose (>3,500 cGy) and low-dose (<2,500 cGy) axial skeletal radiation, and evaluated both sitting (crown rump) height and standing height as a function of age at the time of radiation. Their observations were expressed as standard deviations from the mean and compared to a group of 15,000 normal American-born white children from the San Francisco Bay area. They observed a disporoportionate alteration in sitting height as compared to standing height, which was most marked in those who received high doses (>3,500 cGy) of axial skeletal radiation. This was most marked in those children less than six years of age and those between 11–13 years of age at the time of treatment, both times when bone growth is particularly active. Their studies suffered from a lack of pretreatment or baseline data and from short follow-up. Others have described similar observations to those initially described by Probert and Parker, and some feel that boys are more severely affected than girls [15]. The impact of high-dose, extended field radiation when given to a child of a young age is one of overall reduced height. Figures 2 and 3 demonstrate these radiographic features. Figure 2 shows a chest radiograph 30 years following delivery of 40.0 Gy to a girl of five years of age. It reveals a narrow upper thorax and small clavicles. Figure 3 shows the abdominal pelvic features in the same patient with decreased height of the irradiated vertebrae, sclerosis, and flattening of the acetabula.

In an attempt to better quantitate the severity of growth abnormalities, the

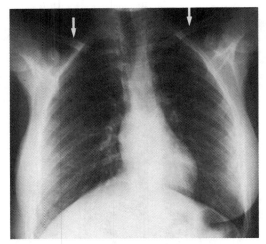

Fig. 2. A chest X-ray of a 30-year-old woman, irradiated to 40.0 Gy total lymphoid irradiation at age five for stage IIIB Hodgkin's disease. While cured of the disease, the sequelae of the radiation are demonstrated by narrowing of the superior thorax, diminution of the bilateral clavicles (arrows), and atrophy of the tissues of the neck and chest.

Stanford investigators evaluated children with Hodgkin's disease in whom pretreatment (baseline) measurements were available, as well as long-term follow-up to age 16 years or to age at cessation of growth. They confirmed that age at the time of treatment, total dose of radiation, and volume treated were all critical parameters with respect to ultimate stature obtained. Their data showed that children less than 13 years of age at the time of treatment were more likely to be impacted by therapy, particularly if they received a high dose (>3,500 cGy) to a large volume (subtotal lymphoid irradiation or total lymphoid irradiation) [16]. Among such a cohort, there was a 5.7% loss of standing height from baseline measurement to final attained stature, which is considered clinically significant in that it exceeds the standard deviation of the mean for nonirradiated control children [16]. The standard deviation in height varies as a

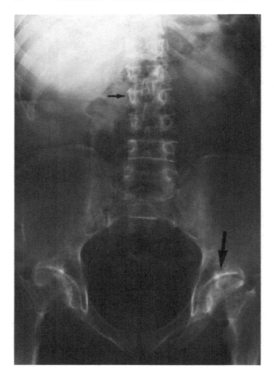

Fig. 3. The abdominal–pelvic bony changes following 40.0 Gy at age five, in the same patient as shown in Figure 2, demonstrates shortened, flattened vertebral bodies (small arrow) and shortening of the femoral necks with sclerotic change (large arrow). These findings have resulted in a shortened overall stature for this 30-year-old woman.

function of age, but in general, ranges between 3.5% and 5%. The variation in standard deviation corresponds to approximately three in. of height in a 5 ft 10 in. individual. The Stanford investigators were unable to demonstrate clinically significant decreases in height among those children 13 years of age or more at the time of treatment, or among children under 13 years of age who received a mantle treatment portal or smaller field (i.e., no subdiaphragmatic radiotherapy). These investigators concluded that when using sitting and standing height measurements to assess bone growth, significant growth abnormalities could *not* be

observed when adolescents or older age children were irradiated. They also concluded that radiation doses <2,500 cGy and small (involved field) volumes do not impair bone growth significantly [16].

PREDICTIVE ASSAYS

An attempt to predict stature loss following skeletal irradiation has been made by Silber et al. [17]. These authors have developed a multiple linear regression model to predict adult stature (MPAS) following irradiation. The model is based upon radiation dose in gray, adjusted for the location of the therapy and attained stature, a femur correction if both acetabula or heads of the femurs were irradiated, gender, and ideal adult stature. The ideal adult stature (IAS) calculation they used was obtained by the Roche-Wainer-Thissen method, which estimates adult stature of a healthy child on the basis of the individual sex, age, stature, weight, and parental stature [18–20]. Thus, in an irradiated patient, stature loss as a result of treatment, represents the difference in the IAS calculation of a healthy individual who never had a diagnosis of cancer and never received radiation, and that calculated by the MPAS based upon the significant variables of radiation dose, field size, and age at the time of treatment. The Silber model was based on 36 children who had either spinal and/or pelvic radiation and 13 nonirradiated children to serve as controls. These authors were unable to confirm that stature velocity, that is, radiation at a period of rapid growth such as adolescence, was a significant factor in impacting ultimate growth disturbance. Moreover, they could not assess the effect of chemotherapy as a radiation enhancer or as an independent variable because of small patient numbers.

The model is intended to serve as a means for clinicians to predict expected stature loss from treatment. We therefore tested its predictive value by applying it to three children with Hodgkin's disease irradiated to a large portion of the spine at a young age. All had the requisite pretreatment data available, and long-term follow-up to demonstrate actual growth attained.

Case 1. NR, an 8-year-old girl found in 1973 to have pathologic stage III mixed cellularity Hodgkin's disease, was treated with total lymphoid irradiation to 44.0 Gy and six cycles of adjuvant MOPP (mustard, oncovin, procarbazine, prednisone) chemotherapy. She remains free of disease with 17 years of follow-up. Her growth patterns are shown in Figure 4. Although only eight years of age when diagnosed, this girl was slightly tall for her age when irradiated. She fell behind in sitting height during her adolescent years, but by age 17–18 she completed her growth at the mean normal for her age. Using the MPAS of Silber, she was predicted to have an ultimate height of 151.3 cm, 9.4 cm shorter than the 160.7 cm she actually achieved.

Case 2. AL, a 10-year-old boy with pathologic stage $III_S A$ nodular sclerosing Hodgkin's disease, was treated on a combined modality protocol utilizing 15.0 Gy subtotal lymphoid irradiation and six cycles of MOPP. At eight years follow-up, he remains free of disease and free of sequelae of treatment. His growth chart is shown in Figure 5, demonstrating that his weight and sitting height were below normal for his age at the time of diagnosis and treatment. His sitting height continued to be at the lower limit of normal throughout his adolescence, but by age 17 his height stabilized at normal levels. We believed this boy would have a normal growth pattern because he received only low doses of irradiation. He was predicted by the MPAS calculation of Silber to have a height of 1.5 cm greater than that which he actually achieved.

Case 3. TB, an 11½-year-old girl with pathologic stage $III_S B$ lymphocyte de-

pleted Hodgkin's disease, was treated in 1970 with 44.0 Gy total lymphoid irradiation and six cycles of MOPP. With 20 years of follow-up, she continues free of disease. Her growth is shown in Figure 6. She was small for her age in sitting height and weight when treated at age 11½ years, but her standing height was above the norm for her age. She has had no growth as measured by sitting or standing height measurements since treatment, and thus has an ultimate height of 160.7

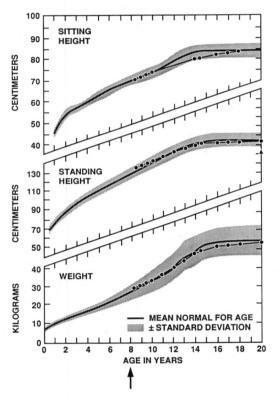

Fig. 4. Sitting height, standing height, and weight for a girl irradiated at age eight for stage III Hodgkin's disease. The arrow demonstrates her age when treated. Despite receiving 44.0 Gy total lymphoid irradiation, her ultimate standing height, sitting height, and weight are at the mean normal for her age, as plotted on standard growth curves of Tanner. The triangle depicts her MPAS, which was calculated to be 9.4 cm shorter than she actually attained.

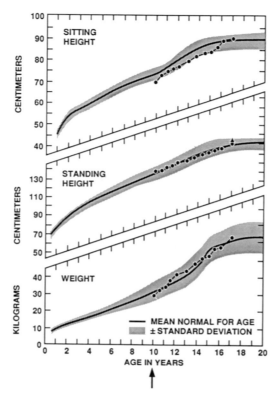

Fig. 5. Sitting height, standing height, and weight for a 10-year-old boy irradiated to 15.0 Gy subtotal lymphoid irradiation for stage III Hodgkin's disease. The arrow demonstrates his age when treated. His ultimate height was within normal limits as predicted by Tanner, although 1.5 cm shorter than predicted by the MPAS model (see triangle).

cm, which is at the lower limit of the standard deviation of the mean for her age. The MPAS predicted her ultimate height to be 157.3 cm or 3.4 cm shorter than she actually attained.

In our experience, the MPAS has not correlated well with actual clinical findings in the two cases shown in Figures 4 and 6, where we anticipated significant growth alterations. This may relate to differences in the control data, or problems with small numbers. However, these three cases do illustrate the difficulties in estab-

lishing an effective predictive assay to quantitate ultimate attained stature, and the large number of variables impacting such an outcome.

SECONDARY MALIGNANT TUMOR

Neoplastic transformation of irradiated bone is the most severe of the observed late sequelae and, fortunately, is a rare occurrence. The most commonly observed benign lesion following radiotherapy is

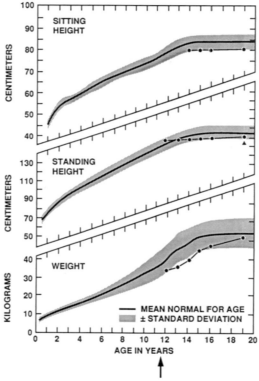

Fig. 6. Sitting height and weight for an 11½-year-old girl irradiated to 44.0 Gy total lymphoid irradiation. Although slightly taller than the Tanner control for her age when treated, she had essentially no standing or sitting height growth after treatment, and ended with an ultimate height of 160.7 cm (one standard deviation below the Tanner mean normal). The MPAS model (triangle) predicted her ultimate height to be 3.4 cm shorter than actually attained.

the osteocartilaginous exostosis, which may occur in any irradiated area. Malignant transformation within a radiation exostosis has not been reported. However, postirradiation soft tissue and bone sarcomas are being observed with increasing frequency as cure rates from childhood malignancies improve and follow-up duration is increased. Orbital and paranasal sinus osteosarcomas among survivors of retinoblastoma were initially explained by the extremely high doses of irradiation and the kilovoltage irradiation used. More recently, it has been understood that there is a genetic predisposition to develop secondary sarcomas among patients with hereditary retinoblastoma, and the retinoblastoma gene on chromosome 13 q 14 has been identified. Approximately one-third of the secondary sarcomas in these patients arise in sites distant to the irradiated field. Furthermore, paranasal sinus sarcoma has been reported among retinoblastoma survivors managed by enucleation alone without radiation. Irradiated babies with nonhereditary retinoblastoma and/or unilateral retinoblastoma do not have an increased risk for the development of these high grade sarcomas. Thus, it appears that the genetic factor plays the major role in malignant second tumor induction among survivors of retinoblastoma. Secondary solid tumors, however, have also been reported among patients cured of Ewing's sarcoma and Hodgkin's disease [21–23]. These tumors have frequently been in patients receiving combined modality treatment, but the relationship to prior radiation therapy cannot be denied.

SOLUTION

The deleterious skeletal effects of radiation can be minimized by adopting certain routines:

1. Always utilize homogeneous, well-collimated megavoltage radiation.

2. Never use orthovoltage in children.

3. Never use high-dose per fraction and high total doses.

4. Treatment volumes need to be determined precisely, and shrinking fields should be employed.

5. Shield growth centers whenever possible.

6. Avoid radiation to sites with inadequate vascular supply or in patients with a history of vascular disease.

There is a major need to develop specific methods to quantitate the degree of skeletal injury, to precisely and accurately relate the dose/volume/age guidelines, and to devise predictive assays so as to advise patients and parents appropriately. These factors then need to be weighed against the efficacy and value of the therapy so rational therapeutic decisions can be determined.

Bone and soft tissue abnormalities from radiation are matters of concern, but their extent has been greatly exaggerated in the past. Serious skeletal injuries can largely be avoided through an awareness of the potential skeletal effects of radiation, and through the use of modern, properly administered radiotherapy.

ACKNOWLEDGMENTS

This study was supported in part by grant CA 34244 from the National Cancer Institute, National Institutes of Health, Bethesda, Maryland.

REFERENCES

1. Perthes G: Uber deb Einfluss der roetgenstrahlen auf epitheliale gewebe, insbesondere aus des carcinom. Arch Klin Chir 51:955, 1903 (cited by Dawson WB, Clin Radiol 19:241–156, 1968).
2. Fosterling K: Uber allgemeine und partielle washstums storungen nach kurz dauernden rontgen bestrahlungen von saugethieren. Arch Klin Chir 81:506, 1906 (cited by Dawson WB, Clin Radiol 29:241–256, 1968).

3. Dalinka MK, Mazzeo V: Complications of radiation therapy. Crit Rev Diagn Imaging 23:236–267, 1984.

4. Berdon WE, Baker DH, Boyer J: Unusual benign and malignant sequelae to childhood radiation therapy. AJR 93:545–556, 1965.

5. Rutherford H, Dodd G: Complications of radiation therapy: Growing bone. Sem Roentgenol 9:15–27, 1974.

6. Sengupta S, Prathup K: Radiation necrosis of the humerus. A report of three cases. Acta Radiol Ther Phys Biol 12:313–320, 1973.

7. Fajardo LF: Locomotive System in Pathology of Radiation Injury. New York: Masson Publishing, 1982, pp 176–185.

8. Rubin P, Casarett GW (eds): Clinical Radiation Pathology (Volume II), Philadelphia: WB Saunders, 1968, pp 518–577.

9. Zeman W, Solomon M: Effects of radiation on striated muscle. In Bergdjis CC (ed): Pathology of Irradiation. Baltimore: Williams and Wilkins, 1971, pp 171–185.

10. Probert JC, Parker BR: The effects of radiation therapy on bone growth. Radiology 114:155–162, 1975.

11. Halperin EC, Kun LE, Constine LS, Tarbell NJ (eds): Pediatric Radiation Oncology. New York: Raven Press, 1989, pp 348–354.

12. Anderson M, Green WT, Messner MB: Growth and predictions of growth in the lower extremities. J Bone Joint Surg 45A:1–14, 1963.

13. Menelaus MB: Correction of leg length discrepancy by epiphysial arrest. J Bone Joint Surg 48B:336–339, 1966.

14. White JW, Stubbins SJ: Growth arrest for equalizing leg lengths. JAMA 126:1146, 1944.

15. Wilimas J, Thompson E, Smith KL: Long-term results of treatment of children and adolescents with Hodgkin's disease. Cancer 46:2123–2125, 1980.

16. Donaldson SS, Kleeberg P, Cox R: Growth abnormalities associated with radiation in children with Hodgkin's disease. Proc Am Soc Clin Oncol 7:224, 1988.

17. Silber JH, Littman PS, Meadows AT: Stature loss following skeletal irradiation for childhood cancer. J Clin Oncol 8:304–312, 1990.

18. Roche AF, Wainer H, Thissen D: Predicting adult stature for individuals. Mong Pediatr 3:1–115, 1975.

19. Roche AF, Wainer H, Thissen D: The RWT method for prediction of adult stature. Pediatrics 56:1026–1033, 1975.

20. Roche AF: Adult stature predictions: A critical review. Acta Med Auxol 16:5–28, 1985.

21. Tucker MA, D'Angio GJ, Boice JD, et al.: Bone sarcomas linked to radiotherapy and chemotherapy in children. N Engl J Med 317:588–593, 1987.

22. Koletsky AJ, Bertino JR, Farber LR, et al.: Second neoplasms in patients with Hodgkin's disease following combined modality therapy: The Yale experience. J Clin Oncol 4:311–317, 1986.

23. Coleman CN, Kaplan HS, Cox R, et al.: Leukemias, non-Hodgkin's lymphomas and solid tumors in patients treated for Hodgkin's disease. Cancer Surv 1:733–744, 1982.

10

Indications for Human Growth Hormone Treatment of Radiation-Induced Growth Hormone Deficiency

S.M. Shalet, M.D., A.L. Ogilvy-Stuart, M.R.C.P., E.C. Crowne, M.R.C.P., and P.E. Clayton, M.D.

Children with brain tumors not directly involving the hypothalamic-pituitary axis, extracranial tumors including nasopharyngeal carcinoma and retinoblastoma, acute lymphoblastic leukemia (ALL) and other leukemias, may develop growth hormone (GH) deficiency as a consequence of external irradiation to the hypothalamic-pituitary axis. The children treated for brain tumors receive higher doses of cranial irradiation than those receiving prophylactic cranial radiation therapy for ALL. Finally, the children with leukemia, who are offered bone marrow transplantation (BMT), may receive total body irradiation (TBI) as part of the preparative treatment to suppress the immune system and eradicate the underlying hematological disorder.

The degree of pituitary hormonal deficit is related to the radiation dose received by the hypothalamic-pituitary axis. Thus, after lower radiation doses, isolated GH deficiency ensues, whereas higher doses may produce panhypopituitarism. The vast majority of the children considered in this review, however, have isolated GH deficiency and thus growth responses to GH therapy are not complicated by other pituitary hormone deficits. Furthermore, the greater the radiation dose, the earlier GH deficiency will occur after treatment. Between two and five years after irradia-tion, 100% of children receiving $\geq$ 3,000 cGy to the hypothalamic-pituitary axis show subnormal GH responses to an insulin tolerance test (ITT), while 35% of those receiving < 3,000 cGy show a normal GH response [1]. Prospective studies including our own, however, concentrate on GH responses to provocative tests, while the speed of onset of physiological GH deficiency following radiation-induced damage remains unknown.

To determine if GH has had a significant impact on growth in children with radiation-induced GH deficiency, the growth velocity during the first year of GH treatment has been compared with the pretreatment growth velocity [2–5]. This will indicate whether there has been a significant short-term improvement in growth rate, but not if there will be a substantial gain in final height. Thus, long-term studies are the most critical. Ideally, these should include an analysis of the final height and gain or loss in stature (SDS) from initiation of GH therapy until the end of growth in children with radiation-induced GH deficiency. These results should then be contrasted with the growth pattern in those who did not receive GH therapy and with the results seen in children with idiopathic isolated GH deficiency treated with GH therapy.

Late Effects of Treatment for Childhood Cancer, pages 71–79 © 1992 Wiley-Liss, Inc.

BRAIN TUMORS

The marked impairment of spinal growth following axial irradiation means that it is inappropriate to compare the growth responses of children who have received cranial irradiation with those receiving craniospinal irradiation. These two groups must be considered separately.

In our Centre the growth response to GH therapy has been studied in 12 children with GH deficiency following cranial irradiation and in 14 children with idiopathic GH deficiency. Before treatment, the cranially irradiated patients had higher standard deviation scores (SDS) for standing height, sitting height and leg length, and less bone age retardation. Both groups started treatment at a similar age (11–12 years) with a similar pretreatment height velocity and peak GH response to standard provocative tests. Growth hormone therapy administered in a schedule of four units intramuscularly three times a week produced a significant and similar increase in height velocity over the first two years of treatment in both groups. At completion of growth, however, cranially irradiated children (N = 7) showed no change in height SDS with GH therapy, compared to marked catch-up growth in the idiopathic GH deficient children (N = 14) (Figs. 1 and 2). Nevertheless, GH enabled cranially irradiated patients to maintain their centile position and to achieve a more acceptable final height than if they had remained untreated.

Children with radiation-induced GH deficiency after craniospinal irradiation who had received GH therapy (CS) were compared with those who remained untreated (NCS) [7]. The mean age at diagnosis of GH deficiency was 11 years in both groups and the duration of GH therapy or clinic review in both the treated and untreated patients was four years. Growth hormone therapy (four units

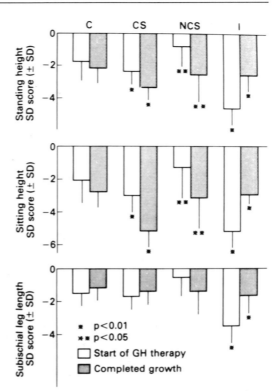

Fig. 1. Mean standing height, sitting height, and leg length SD scores at the start of GH therapy/clinic review, and at completed growth in GH-treated cranially irradiated (C), craniospinal irradiated (CS), idiopathic GH-deficient children (I), and in an untreated group of craniospinal irradiated children (NCS).

three times a week) produced a significant increase in height velocity over the first three years in the treated group, with a mean first year increment of 3 cm. Patients treated to completion of growth (N = 8) showed a significant increase in leg length SD (▲ SDS, +0.2) compared to that of the untreated group (N = 7) (▲ SDS, −0.9). Sitting height SDS decreased equally in both groups (by −1.7 for the treated and −2.2 for the untreated), indicating that GH therapy had not ameliorated the impairment of spinal growth caused by spinal irradiation (Figs. 1 and 2).

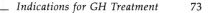

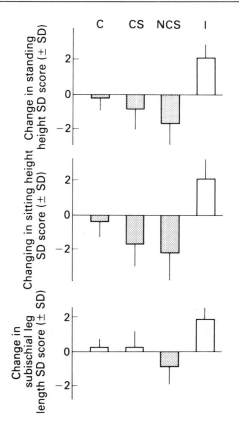

Fig. 2. Mean change in SD scores for standing height, sitting height, and leg length over the period of GH therapy/clinic review in GH-treated cranial irradiation (C), craniospinal irradiated (CS), idiopathic GH-deficient children (I), and in an untreated group of craniospinal irradiated children (NCS).

At completion of GH therapy, there was a mean decrease in standing height SDS of 0.9 in the treated group, but a decrease of 1.7 in those not treated with GH. Thus, although GH therapy failed to induce "catch-up" growth in craniospinal irradiated patients, it did prevent further loss in achieving adult stature, with a mean final height SDS of −3.4 in treated patients [7].

Our studies indicated that GH therapy was of benefit in children with radiation-induced GH deficiency. However, the height gained, or rather the "height loss,"

that had been prevented was disappointingly small and much less than that seen in GH-treated children with idiopathic GH deficiency.

There are a number of factors responsible for the suboptimal growth response. These include spinal irradiation, precocious or early puberty, the excessively long time interval between the development of radiation-induced GH deficiency and the initiation of GH therapy, and the inadequacy of the GH schedule used in our early studies.

Spinal irradiation may have a profound effect on spinal growth [8]. The younger the child at the time of irradiation, the greater the subsequent skeletal disproportion, which is only seen to its full extent once puberty is completed [9]. A conservative estimate of the eventual loss in height ranges from 9 cm if irradiated at one year to 5.5 cm at 10 years of age. Early or precocious puberty has been reported in some children who have received cranial irradiation [3,10]. In a group of irradiated children aged 1–13 years, we have shown that the age at pubertal onset is positively correlated to the age at irradiation (Fig. 3). It is therefore the youngest at irradiation who are likely to have the most profound disturbances in the timing of puberty and in whom the clinical consequences will be most readily apparent. The mean age at puberty of these children is similar to that of normal children. In the presence of GH deficiency, however, which is usually associated with delay in the onset of puberty, it is abnormal.

A disturbance in pubertal timing in females rather than males has also been reported in those receiving prophylactic cranial irradiation for ALL [11,12]. These females entered puberty early and as a group, the age at menarche was positively correlated with the age at irradiation. Therefore, we examined the relationship between the onset of puberty and age at

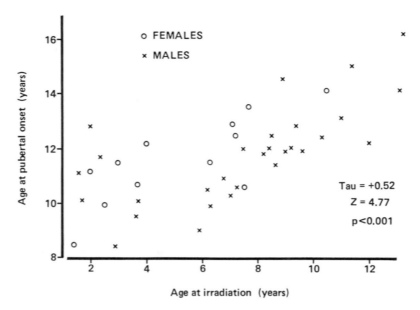

Fig. 3. Relationship between age at irradiation and age at pubertal onset in 41 children who received cranial/craniospinal irradiation for a brain tumor or prophylactic CNS irradiation for ALL.

irradiation in a group of boys and girls treated for either a brain tumor or ALL who received their cranial irradiation at least three years before the normal age of pubertal onset [13].

The mean chronological age at pubertal onset in the males was early at 11.1 ± 1.4 and significantly different from normal (mean 11.8 years). The females entered puberty at a normal chronological age of 11.4 ± 1.4 years. The mean bone age at pubertal onset was early in both the males (10.3 ± 1.9 years) and females (9.6 ± 1.0 years). The relationship between irradiation and pubertal onset followed a linear correlation for females: those irradiated at the youngest ages had the earliest pubertal onset. In contrast the relationship for males was more complex. Pubertal onset was earliest for those irradiated between the ages of three and six years. No relationship was apparent between irradiation dosage across the range 2,400–4,750 cGy and the age at pubertal onset for the whole group. The difference in pubertal timing for males and females is unexplained. However, a shift in the onset of puberty was not restricted to females.

The impact of early puberty in a child with radiation-induced growth failure is to foreshorten the time available for GH therapy. Consequently, at our own and other centres, some of these children are treated with a combination of a GnRH analog and GH therapy. It is relatively easy to halt the progression in pubertal development but it is too early to analyze the impact of this approach on final height.

In the studies reported by Clayton et al. [6,7], GH therapy was initiated in a child only if biochemical evidence of GH deficiency was associated with a poor growth velocity (<25th centile) established over at least one year. Thus, the mean time interval between irradiation and starting GH therapy was 5.5–6.7 years in the two studies. This time interval is too long and means that some growth potential is lost irrevocably. Since 1987 children with radiation-induced GH deficiency have been treated much earlier after cranial irradiation than previously. This is illustrated in Figs. 4 and 5 where it can be seen that the "post-1987" children have a much better growth velocity in the pre-GH treatment year than the "pre-1987" children. The mean time interval between irradiation and initiation of GH therapy in the "post-1987" children was 3.7 years.

For many years the standard GH schedule for the treatment of GH deficient children in the United Kingdom was four units administered three times a week irrespective of size. Now that there are abundant supplies of GH, it has become clear that the frequency of administration and the dose of GH are critical factors that influence the growth response. The children reported by Clayton et al. received a total weekly mean GH dose of 0.4

units/kg in three injections a week [6,7]. Our current GH schedule is 0.5 units/kg/week administered by daily injection. The growth velocity of our GH-deficient children was 7.4 cm in those cranially irradiated and 6.2 cm in those craniospinally irradiated during the first year of GH therapy [6,7]. Recently, Lannering and Albertsson-Wikland [5] reported the growth response to GH therapy in 15 children with radiation-induced GH deficiency following treatment for a brain tumor. Four of the 15 children had received craniospinal irradiation. The mean pretreatment growth velocity of the Swedish children was similar to that of the children studied by Clayton et al. [6,7]. The mean growth velocity during the first year of GH therapy was 8.2 cm, which significantly exceeded that seen in the Manchester children. Furthermore, the improved growth velocity results were maintained

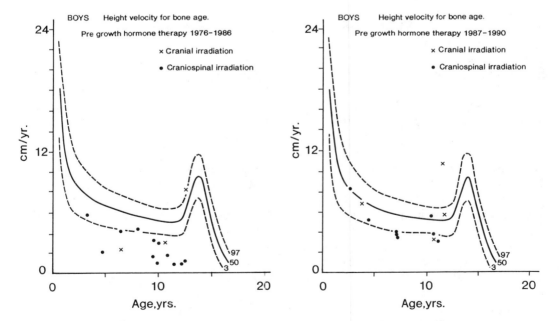

Fig. 4. Pre-GH treatment growth velocity in boys with radiation-induced GH deficiency following the treatment of a brain tumor. All of these boys were prescribed GH before 1987.

Fig. 5. Pre-GH treatment growth velocity in boys with radiation GH deficiency following the treatment of a brain tumor. All of these boys were prescribed GH after January 1987.

during the second year of GH therapy. In the Swedish study the children received 0.7 units/kg/week administered by daily injection.

CLINICAL PRACTICE

Our clinical criteria for whom to treat and when to initiate GH therapy have continued to evolve in the interval since the first children with radiation-induced GH deficiency treated with GH therapy reached their final height.

The chances of recurrence of a brain tumor are greatest within two years of the primary treatment of the tumor. There is no evidence that treatment with GH increases the risk of recurrence of a brain tumor in children with radiation-induced GH deficiency [14]. A reasonable approach therefore would be to initiate treatment with GH two years after irradiation of all children with brain tumors treated by standard radiation schedules, which included a dose to the hypothalamic-pituitary axis in excess of 3,000 cGy. At this time they would no longer be receiving cytotoxic chemotherapy, the chance of recurrence of a tumor is low and it is established that most, if not all, will be GH-deficient by this time. This policy would be independent of the child's growth rate (Figs. 4 and 5) and would not require routine tests of GH secretion.

Many of the children irradiated for a brain tumor, who receive a dose of 2,500–3,000 cGy will be GH-deficient two years after primary treatment. Thus, these children undergo standard provocative tests of GH release at two years and if the results are abnormal they receive GH therapy. If GH secretion appears normal and the growth rate is appropriate for bone age and pubertal status, then growth is observed and the GH stimulation tests are repeated annually. However, if the growth rate is subnormal in the presence of normal GH responses to pharmacological stimuli, a combination that is very un-

usual in our centre, then radiation-induced GH neurosecretory dysfunction may be a possible explanation. The alternative approaches would be either an appraisal of physiological GH secretion, such as a 24-hr profile, or an empirical trial of GH therapy.

These guidelines assume that in craniospinal irradiated children, growth is assessed by leg length velocity, and that other causes of poor growth, such as radiation-induced hypothyroidism, recurrent tumor, and malnutrition have been excluded.

The principle behind the policy is to administer GH therapy earlier in this group of children and thereby improve their ultimate height prognosis.

ACUTE LYMPHOBLASTIC LEUKEMIA

Much confusion and controversy have been generated over the growth patterns and GH requirements of the child with acute lymphoblastic leukemia treated with prophylactic cranial irradiation and combination cytotoxic chemotherapy for several years. Some groups have found no adverse effect on final height, while other groups (including our own) have noted a modest adverse effect on growth [15]. As final height is unknown in most of the children, however, the possibility of impaired pubertal growth may mean that final height loss is substantial in a proportion of children. Finally, Kirk et al. [16] studied children with acute lymphoblastic leukemia and found a much greater retardation of growth. An analysis of the radiation schedules and chemotherapy protocols used in the different centers has led to some understanding of the reasons for the differences in height loss observed among groups.

There is in vitro evidence that cytotoxic chemotherapy may affect growth mechanisms and in vivo evidence of an effect on growth [15,16]. In the child with acute lymphoblastic leukemia, the duration and nature of the combination cytotoxic chemotherapy will influence the growth prognosis. The effects of cytotoxic chemotherapy with the regimens used in the United Kingdom are likely to be minor, but more intense drug regimens have had a profound impact on growth [16]. Children irradiated prophylactically for acute lymphoblastic leukemia rather than for a brain tumor tend to receive a lower radiation dose to the hypothalamic–pituitary axis. Most of the growth studies have been carried out in children who received a total cranial radiation dose of 2,400–2,500 cGy. The incidence of GH deficiency in such children will depend on the number of fractions, fraction size, and duration of the radiation schedule.

For a number of reasons, the demand for treatment with GH is more difficult to predict after treatment for acute lymphoblastic leukemia than after a brain tumor. The dissimilar growth patterns in children with acute lymphoblastic leukemia studied by different groups have already been discussed. Radiation induced GH deficiency is common in children with severe growth retardation, even though cytotoxic chemotherapy is a serious adverse factor [16]. It is appropriate therefore that most of these children be offered treatment with GH. However, only a minority of children with acute lymphoblastic leukemia in our Manchester center have been treated with GH. In them, chemotherapy appears to be only a minor adverse factor. The clinical dilemma is how to identify the few who should receive treatment. We have suggested that a therapeutic trial of GH should be offered to those children who are GH deficient and who are below the tenth centile or whose growth rate is persistently poor after completion of cytotoxic chemotherapy. It should be understood, however, that this is an arbitrary definition of GH requirement.

Moell et al. [11] have studied the growth patterns of children with acute lympho-

blastic leukemia during different phases of childhood. The girls lost very little standing height SD score during prepubertal life, as in other studies, but had an attenuated pubertal growth spurt. The contribution of GH deficiency to the disturbed pubertal growth is under investigation. Also under study is the effect of treatment with GH to improve it, with or without the addition of a gonadotrophin releasing hormone analog to delay the rather early pubertal onset in some of the girls.

Since 1980, the total dose of cranial irradiation for ALL has been reduced to 1,800 cGy. A pilot study of 24-hr GH secretion in 19 ALL children who received 1,800-cGy cranial irradiation and in 17 normal children has been completed recently [17]. The mean area under the GH curve (AUC) in the prepubertal ALL children was not significantly different from that of the normal prepubertal children. However, there was a significant increase in GH AUC between the prepubertal and pubertal normal children but not in those who had received 1,800 cGy. These preliminary results suggest that after the lower dose of cranial irradiation, prepubertal growth and GH secretion will be normal in the vast majority of children but that growth and GH secretion during puberty will be attenuated in a significant proportion.

Thus, after 1,800 cGy, GH therapy may need to be considered for ALL children around the age of onset of puberty if their current standing height lies below the tenth centile. This is a very tentative suggestion as detailed growth data are required to define the frequency with which the growth spurt is attenuated, and the severity of the height loss in those affected.

TOTAL BODY IRRADIATION

Marrow transplantation has become a lifesaving procedure for an increasing number of children and young adults with either nonmalignant or malignant hematological disorders, in particular leukemia. Follow-up studies evaluating growth and development have shown that the delayed effects are related to the regimen used for preparation for marrow transplantation. Few endocrine abnormalities have been observed after regimens containing only high doses of cyclophosphamide, but growth disturbance and multiple endocrine abnormalities have been seen after regimens that include TBI [18].

Total body irradiation has been given in single-dose exposures of 750–1,000 cGy, and more recently, in fractionated exposures of total doses ranging from 1,200 to 1,575 cGy given over a period of three–seven days. Severe growth disturbance is common and may be caused by various etiological factors including GH deficiency, thyroid dysfunction, radiation-induced impairment of skeletal growth, or graft versus host disease and its treatment. Growth hormone deficiency may occur even if the child has not received prophylactic cranial irradiation previously [19].

Following TBI (1,000–1,320 cGy in 5–6 fractions over three days) in adults, GH secretion, assessed by the GH response to an ITT, appears intact [20]. It is unclear whether the GH deficiency following TBI described by Borgstrom and Bolme [19] reflects a greater radiosensitivity of the hypothalamus in children compared to adults. An alternative explanation for these different findings might be the TBI radiation schedules. The children studied by Borgstrom and Bolme [19] received 1,000 cGy in a single fraction.

There is a desperate need for more information on the impact of single and fractionated courses of 1,000–1,300 cGy TBI on the incidence of GH deficiency, GH neurosecretory dysfunction, speed of onset of GH deficiency, and cartilage growth. Without such information the growth problems of this group of patients remain among the most difficult encountered in clinical practice. Once graft versus host disease and hypothyroidism have been excluded in a child growing poorly after TBI, standard provocative tests of GH secretion are required. Growth hormone therapy should be offered if the GH responses are found to be subnormal. Questions remain when GH responses are normal: Is the child growing slowly because of poor cartilage growth or GH neurosecretory dysfunction? Should a 24-hr GH profile be performed to try and establish the latter diagnosis or should the child receive an empirical trial of GH therapy? If GH therapy is instituted, what is the optimum schedule in the likely presence of GH deficiency and radiation-induced skeletal dysplasia?

CONCLUSIONS

After 15 years of research we now have reasonably well-founded therapeutic strategies for the children with radiation-induced GH deficiency following the treatment of brain tumors in childhood. The study of growth patterns in the children treated for ALL has illustrated potential impact of certain combinations of cytotoxic drugs on growth. Furthermore, it has emphasized that the potential need for GH therapy is greatest when there are multiple adverse factors affecting growth including GH deficiency!

Finally, review of the few studies of growth in children who have received TBI indicates enormous need for more information.

REFERENCES

1. Clayton PE, Shalet SM: Dose-dependency of time of onset of radiation-induced growth hormone deficiency. J Pediatr 118:226–228, 1991.
2. Shalet SM, Whitehead E, Chapman AJ, Beardwell CG: The effects of growth hormone therapy in children with radiation-induced growth hormone deficiency. Acta Paediatr Scand 70: 81–85, 1981.

3. Winter RJ, Green OC: Irradiation-induced growth hormone deficiency: blunted growth response and accelerated skeletal maturation to growth hormone therapy. J Pediatr 4:609–612, 1985.

4. Romshe CA, Zipf WB, Miser A, Miser J, Newton WA: Evaluation of growth hormone release and human growth hormone treatment in children with cranial irradiation associated short stature. J Pediatr 104:177–181, 1984.

5. Lannering B, Albertsson-Wikland: Improved growth response to GH treatment in irradiated children. Acta Paediatr Scand 78:562–567, 1989.

6. Clayton PE, Shalet SM, Price DA: Growth response to growth hormone therapy following cranial irradiation. Eur J Pediatr 147:593–596, 1988a.

7. Clayton PE, Shalet SM, Price DA: Growth response to growth hormone therapy following craniospinal irradiation. Eur J Pediatr 147:597–601, 1988b.

8. Shalet SM, Gibson B, Swindell R, Pearson D: Effect of spinal irradiation on growth. Arch Dis Child 62:461–464, 1987.

9. Clayton PE, Shalet SM: The evolution of spinal growth after irradiation. J Clin Oncol 3:220–222, 1991.

10. Brauner R, Czernichow P, Rappaport R: Precocious puberty after hypothalamic and pituitary irradiation in young children. N Eng J Med 311:920, 1984.

11. Moell C, Garwicz S, Westgren V, Wiebe T: Disturbed pubertal growth in girls treated for acute lymphoblastic leukemia. Pediatr Hematol Oncol 4:1–5, 1987.

12. Leiper AD, Stanhope R, Kitching P, Chessells JM: Precocious and premature puberty associated with treatment of acute lymphoblastic leukemia. Arch Dis Child 62:1107–1112, 1987.

13. Clayton PE, Shalet SM, Gattamaneni HR: Does cranial irradiation cause early puberty? J Endocrin (Suppl) 117:56A, 1988.

14. Clayton PE, Shalet SM, Gattamaneni HR, Price DA: Does growth hormone cause relapse of brain tumors? Lancet 1:1711–1713, 1987.

15. Clayton PE, Shalet SM, Morris-Jones PH, Price DA: Growth in children treated for acute lymphoblastic leukemia. Lancet 1:460–462, 1988c.

16. Kirk JA, Ragupathy P, Stevens MM, Cowell CT, Menser MA, Bergin M, Tink A, Vines RH, Silink M: Growth failure and growth hormone deficiency after treatment for acute lymphoblastic leukemia. Lancet 1:190–193, 1987.

17. Crowne EC, Wallace WHB, Moore C, Ogilvy-Stuart AL, Shalet SM, Morris-Jones PH: Pubertal rise in spontaneous growth hormone (GH) secretion is attenuated by low dose irradiation. J Clin Oncol (in press).

18. Sanders JE, Buckner CD, Sullivan KM, Doney K, Appelbaum F, Witherspoon R, Storb R, Thomas ED: Growth and development in children after bone marrow transplantation. Hormone Res 30:92–97, 1988.

19. Borgstrom B, Bolme P: Growth and growth hormone in children after bone marrow transplantation. Hormone Res 30:98–100, 1988.

20. Littley MD, Shalet SM, Morgenstern GR, Deakin DP: Endocrine and reproductive dysfunction following fractionated total body irradiation in adults. Q J Med 287:265–274, 1991.

11

Reproductive Physiology

Stephen M. Shalet, M.D., and W.H.B. Wallace, M.R.C.P.

Puberty represents the transitional period between childhood and adult life during which the adolescent growth spurt occurs, secondary sexual characteristics appear, and the capacity for fertility is achieved. The past two decades have witnessed a phenomenal increase in our understanding of the processes that underlie the ontogeny of the hypothalamic-pituitary-gonadal axis, although many questions still remain to be answered. The sequence of events that characterize pubertal maturation can be viewed as part of a continuum extending from sexual differentiation and the development of a functional hypothalamic-pituitary-gonadal axis in the fetus through puberty to the attainment of complete sexual maturation and fertility. The essential component parts of the reproductive system are the arcuate nucleus of the medial basal hypothalamus, the gonadotroph cells located in the anterior pituitary, and the male (testis) or female (ovary) gonads.

The gonadotrophin releasing hormone (GnRH) neurosecretory neurones located in the arcuate nucleus translate neural signals into a chemical signal, the decapeptide GnRH, which is released episodically from axon terminals at the median eminence into the hypothalamic-hypophyseal portal capillary plexus. The pituitary gonadotroph cells in response to episodic stimulation from GnRH release the glycoprotein gonadotrophins luteinising hormone (LH) and follicle stimulating hormone (FSH) into the systemic circula-

tion. In the mature male, LH acts predominantly on the Leydig cells of the testis to produce testosterone, and FSH binds to receptors on the Sertoli cell membrane to promote protein synthetic activity and, with testosterone, facilitate spermatogenesis. In the mature female, appropriate gonadotrophin secretion is required to establish a regular menstrual cycle.

Apart from sex steroid production, it is now clear that both the testes and the ovaries secrete a nonsteroidal product, inhibin, that inhibits the secretion of FSH by the pituitary gland and, to a lesser extent, LH as well. Inhibin is a large glycoprotein made up of two subunits, α and β, joined by disulfide bonds. It has structural homology to transforming growth factor beta, which has led to speculation that inhibin could function as a local growth factor in its tissues of origin.

Inhibin suppresses the secretion of FSH in animals leading to the inhibition of ovulation in the female. Whether it suppresses spermatogenesis is unknown. Gonadal secretion account for most, if not all, circulating inhibin except during pregnancy when the placenta is the source. Serum inhibin concentrations measured by radioimmunoassay, become undetectable after castration in both sexes. Inhibin comes from the granulosa cells in females and is under the control of FSH. In males, inhibin is produced by the Sertoli cells under the control of FSH; however, LH also stimulates its secretion either through an indirect effect on the Sertoli cells or

Late Effects of Treatment for Childhood Cancer, pages 81–88 © 1992 Wiley-Liss, Inc.

through the production of inhibin by the Leydig cells. Serum inhibin levels increase with gonadal maturation during puberty [1] and also during the administration of gonadotrophins to patients with gonadotrophin deficiency. These findings have led to the suggestion that the measurement of serum inhibin may be useful in assessing reproductive capability in a variety of clinical situations.

It has been proposed that the hypothalamic-pituitary-gonadal axis in the human differentiates and functions during fetal life and early infancy [2]. Thereafter, it is suppressed to a low level of activity for almost a decade during childhood before the onset of puberty. Puberty represents not the initiation of pulsatile secretion of GnRH, but the reactivation of the GnRH neurosecretory neurones in the arcuate nucleus after a period of relative quiescence during childhood. Experimental and clinical evidence support the hypothesis that the central nervous system (CNS), not the pituitary gland or gonads, exerts the major restraint on the onset of puberty. This inhibition is mediated through the suppression of GnRH synthesis and its episodic secretion.

The studies of Knobil [3] in the rhesus monkey established the importance of the episodic mode of GnRH secretion. In monkeys with hypothalamic lesions, intermittent administration of exogenous GnRH pulses restored gonadotrophin secretion. By contrast, continuous, nonpulsatile, GnRH administration inhibited gonadotrophin secretion by desensitization of GnRH receptors to the pituitary gonadotrophs. Several groups subsequently have induced the normal endocrinology and harmony of pubertal development in children with delayed or arrested puberty resulting from gonadotrophin deficiency using low-dose intermittent GnRH therapy [4].

The hypothalamic-pituitary gonadotrophin axis in the human is functional during early fetal life [5]. The human fetal pituitary gland can synthesize and store FSH and LH by 10 weeks of gestation and can secrete these hormones by 11 weeks gestation. The pattern of secretion is pulsatile and is mediated by an active fetal GnRH pulse generator. After mid-gestation, there is a decline in serum and pituitary FSH and LH levels, which persists to term. The inhibition of fetal hypothalamic GnRH secretion is mediated by two mechanisms, of which the dominant is the maturation of sex steroid mediated negative feedback. Intrinsic CNS suppression appears less important at this stage.

In early infancy after 12 days of age, the hypothalamic GnRH pulse generator becomes active resulting in intermittent FSH and LH secretion. Plasma testosterone values in the male infant increase to reach peak values, in the pubertal range, at 6–15 weeks and then decline by six months. In the female infant, episodic FSH and LH secretion persists until about 12 months of age and is associated with elevated oestradiol levels. The LH pattern of secretion is similar in males and females in infancy, but there is a striking difference in FSH secretion. A significantly greater rise in FSH occurs in females and may persist for up to two years [6]. The reason for this sex difference in FSH secretion in infancy is unclear, but may represent a more active GnRH pulse generator in the female.

Increased FSH and LH secretion in the human fetus and during infancy is followed by a quiescent period of approximately 10 years during which the reproductive endocrine system appears relatively inactive.

Two mechanisms have been postulated to explain the prepubertal restraint exerted on gonadotrophin secretion. First is a sex steroid-dependent negative feedback mechanism. Second is a sex steroid-independent mechanism dependent on intrinsic CNS inhibitory influences.

There is good evidence for a highly sensitive sex steroid-dependent negative feedback mechanism operating in prepu-

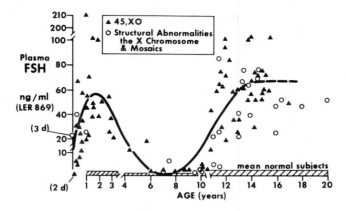

Fig. 1. Change in the pattern of the plasma concentration of FSH with age in 58 patients with the syndrome of gonadal dysgenesis. Triangles designate patients with the 45,X karyotype. Circles indicate Turner syndrome patients with X chromosome mosaicism and/or structural abnormalities of the X chromosome. The solid line represents a regression line of best fit. The hatched area indicates the mean plasma values in normal females [7].

bertal children. Profile studies during this quiescent period have detected low levels of episodic FSH and LH secreted in a circadian pattern. Children with gonadal dysgenesis or congenital anorchia secrete increased amounts of FSH and LH in comparison to normal children (Figs. 1 and 2) and show increased gonadotrophin responses to GnRH [7,8]. These studies indicate that the low levels of sex steroid present in the prepubertal child are capable of inhibiting gonadotrophin secretion.

The diphasic pattern of FSH and LH secretion from infancy through puberty (Figs. 1 and 2) present in both normal and agonadal children cannot, however, be completely explained by a sex steroid-dependent negative feedback mechanism. In children with gonadal dysgenesis, gonadotrophin values are strikingly elevated

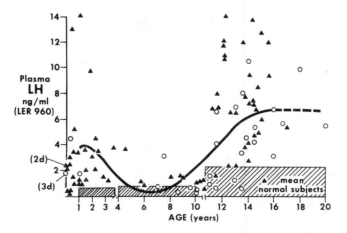

Fig. 2. Change in the pattern of plasma concentrations of LH with age in 58 patients with the syndrome of gonadal dysgenesis (symbols are the same as in Fig. 1) [7].

in infancy and at puberty, but during the prepubertal mid-childhood quiescent period, there is a marked fall in gonadotrophin secretion to levels similar to those found in normal children. This fall in gonadotrophin secretion is independent of gonadal sex steroid and is believed to result from the activity of an intrinsic CNS inhibitory mechanism. This sex steroid independent inhibition located in the CNS appears to be the dominant factor in the suppression of gonadotrophin synthesis and secretion in the prepubertal child. The precise nature and location of this intrinsic CNS inhibitory system remains unclear.

Puberty results from the reactivation of the suppressed GnRH pulse generator associated with increased amplitude and frequency of GnRH secretion, increased gonadotrophin secretion and gonadal maturation. It is likely that in children with central precocious puberty resulting from a hypothalamic neoplasm (or a wide range of CNS lesions including hydrocephalus and cranial irradiation), the lesion destroys the inhibitory neural pathways that have previously suppressed the GnRH pulse generator. Bilateral posterior hypothalamic lesions in female rhesus monkeys resulted in the rapid induction of pubertal maturation, menarche, and ovulation [9], whereas anterior hypothalamic lesions did not advance pubertal development. This experiment points to an intrinsic CNS inhibitory influence present in the posterior hypothalamic region at least in the female rhesus monkey although interpretation of these studies remains controversial.

The specific mechanisms involved in the timing of the onset of puberty in the human are not well understood. There has been a secular trend towards an earlier menarche in girls, and puberty in boys, in Europe and the United States [10]. This progressive decline in the age at puberty is thought to reflect improved socioeconomic standards, general health, and nutrition. Over the last 20 years, there is evidence that this trend has slowed or ceased in developed countries. Nutritional factors and body composition clearly have an important effect on the timing of puberty as evidenced by the earlier age of menarche in moderately obese girls and the delay in the onset of puberty in states of malnutrition or chronic illness [11]. Physical states in girls associated with decreased body fat (e.g., anorexia nervosa, voluntary weight loss, and intensive physical training) are all associated with amenorrhea. The possibility remains that some alteration of body metabolism involving the ratio of fat to lean body mass may affect the intrinsic CNS restraint of pubertal onset.

Tumors of the pineal gland have been associated with precocious puberty in humans, and melatonin secretion from the pineal plays a role in the regulation of reproductive function in seasonally breeding animals [12]. Silman et al. [13] reported a fall in the daytime concentration of melatonin in boys in early puberty, but not in girls. These and other studies led to speculation that the pineal gland, through melatonin secretion, may exert a suppressive effect on the onset of puberty in the human. However, Lenko et al. [14] were unable to confirm the original findings of Silman et al. [13] in a large study of 162 Geneva school children. They found no clear relationship between melatonin concentration and pubertal stage for boys or girls, and concluded that the onset of puberty is not associated with a fall in melatonin secretion. Furthermore, it is now recognized that precocious puberty in association with tumors in the pineal region is usually associated with the secretion of human chorionic gonadotrophin (HCG) [15].

Adrenarche is a maturational change in adrenal function that causes increased secretion of adrenal androgens. The predominant androgens secreted are dehydroepiandrosterone (DHA), DHA sulfate (DHAS), and androstenedione. Adrenarche precedes the onset of puberty by about two years and correlates with the appearance of the adrenal zona reticularis. Adrenal androgens are largely responsible for the appearance of pubic and axillary hair in the female. Normal puberty comprises both adrenarche and maturation of the hypothalamic-pituitary-gonadal axis (gonadarche), however, each process can occur independently in certain pathological situations. A normal onset of puberty occurs in patients with childhood Addison's disease and with premature adrenarche [16,17]. Current evidence suggests that normal levels of adrenal androgens do not exert a major effect on the timing of the onset of puberty.

The onset of puberty in the human is characterized biochemically by the presence of sleep-entrained LH secretion [18]. It is likely that this process is due to an amplification of preexisting low amplitude pulses of GnRH. Wu et al. [19] have recently studied the overnight pattern of pulsatile LH secretion in prepubertal and early pubertal boys using a highly sensitive monoclonal antibody-based immunoradiometric assay. The study cohort were classified retrospectively according to their subsequent clinical course as prepubertal (N = 14), peripubertal (N = 11), or pubertal (N = 5). The patterns of pulsatile LH secretion were compared among the patient groups. The study confirmed that LH pulses are detectable in some prepubertal subjects, and demonstrated that the clinical onset of puberty was preceded by an increase in the frequency of nocturnal pulsatile LH secretion [20]. This implies that GnRH frequency modulation plays an important part in the early pubertal activation of pituitary-gonadal function in the human.

The mean age at the onset of puberty is 11.2 years in girls and 11.4 years in boys. The acquisition of secondary sex characteristics before eight years in girls and nine years in boys constitutes precocious pubertal development. Similarly, children with no signs of puberty by 14 years require specialist assessment. The onset of puberty in girls is usually manifested by breast budding and in boys by enlargement of the testes to a volume of four ml as measured using an orchidometer. The onset of the adolescent growth spurt has a fixed relationship to the stage of pubertal development in both boys and girls. As breast development begins in girls, the growth rate increases to reach a peak at Tanner stage three breast development. When Tanner stage four breast development is reached, menarche occurs and the growth rate declines. The prepubertal growth rate in boys in maintained during the early stages of genital and pubic hair development until a testicular volume of 10 ml is attained; then the growth rate rises. Normal puberty is characterized by the sequential acquisition of secondary sexual characteristics associated with a pubertal growth spurt at an appropriate time.

During the first two years postmenarche, as many as 55–90% of cycles are anovulatory. The explanation of the anovulatory cycles remains speculative. The stimulatory action of oestradiol on gonadotrophin release has not been demonstrated in normal prepubertal or early pubertal children. Thus, positive feedback as part of the normal pubertal process is a late maturational event and possibly does not occur before midpuberty in normal girls. In the light of evidence that positive feedback does not require an increase in GnRH pulse frequency or amplitude and can occur by direct action on the GnRH-primed pituitary gland, the principal limiting step appears to be the pubertal ovary and its capacity to provide sufficient output of oestradiol to induce a gonadotrophin surge.

INFLUENCE OF RADIATION AND CHEMOTHERAPY DURING CHILDHOOD ON THE REPRODUCTIVE AXIS

It is believed that cranial irradiation may damage the intrinsic CNS inhibitory mechanism that restrains GnRH secretion. Early or precocious puberty may thus occur following cranial irradiation for a brain tumor or administered prophylactically as part of the treatment of children with acute lymphoblastic leukemia.

Central precocious puberty may be treated by continued administration of a GnRH agonist analog, which leads to decreased gonadotrophin responsiveness, a fall in circulating FSH and LH levels, decreased gonadal steroids, and a halting or regression of sexual maturation.

Higher radiation doses to the head may result in gonadotrophin deficiency. This is usually a consequence of GnRH deficiency as the hypothalamus is more radiosensitive than the pituitary. The gonadotrophin deficiency could be treated by intermittent pulsatile GnRH therapy providing the pituitary gonadotrophs have not also been damaged by the irradiation. However, in practice, it is far easier to induce pubertal development with sex steroids.

Both irradiation and cytotoxic chemotherapy may damage the gonad directly [22]. The testis and the germinal epithelium in particular are more vulnerable to cytotoxic damage. Just as seen in the girls with Turner's syndrome (Figs. 1 and 2), it is frequently impossible to detect biochemically cytotoxic-induced gonadal damage during prepubertal life (Fig. 3). Abnormally elevated gonadotrophin levels occur only when the child has reached an age at which the onset of puberty would have

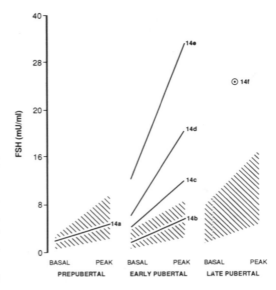

Fig. 3. Basal and peak FSH concentrations after GnRH in a boy treated with multiple courses of MOPP for Hodgkin's disease between the ages of 6 and 9 years. The GnRH tests were performed at: a) 1 year, b) 1.5 years, c) 1.7 years, d) 2 years, e) 3 years after completion of treatment, and f) is the basal FSH level five years posttreatment. Normal ranges of values for each pubertal stage are shown (shaded areas). Note that the basal and stimulated FSH levels remain normal until 1.7 years after completion of chemotherapy despite the fact that the testicular damage will have occurred at the time chemotherapy was administered. This illustrates the unreliability of FSH estimations in predicting testicular damage in prepubertal and peripubertal boys.

been expected [23–25]. The use of more sensitive gonadotrophin assays may, however, detect gonadal damage at a much earlier age in future studies [26].

REFERENCES

1. Burger HG, Maclachlan RI, Bangah M, Quigg H, Findlay JK, Robertson DM, de Kretser DM, Warne GL, Werther GA, Hudson IL, Cook JJ, Fielder R, Greco S, Yong ABW, Smith P: Serum inhibin concentrations rise throughout normal male and female puberty. J Clin Endocrinol Metab 67:689–694, 1988.
2. Grumbach MM, Kaplan SL: The neuroendocrinology of human puberty: An ontogenetic

perspective. In Grumbach MM, Sizonenko PC, Aubert ML (eds): Control of the Onset of Puberty. Maryland: Williams and Wilkins, 1990, pp 1–68.

3. Knobil E: Patterns of hypophysiotropic signals and gonadotrophin secretion in the rhesus monkey. Biol Reprod 24:44–49, 1981.

4. Stanhope R, Brook CGD, Pringle CJ, Adams J, Jacobs HS: Induction of puberty by pulsatile gonadotrophin releasing hormone. Lancet: 552–555, 1987.

5. Gluckman PD, Grumbach MM, Kaplan SL: The human fetal hypothalamus and pituitary gland; the maturation of neuroendocrine mechanisms controlling the secretion of fetal pituitary growth hormone, prolactin, gonadotrophin, and adrenocorticotrophin-related peptides. In Tulchinsky D, Ryan KJ (eds): Maternal-Fetal Endocrinology. Philadelphia: WB Saunders, 1980, pp 196–232.

6. Waldhauser F, Weinbenbacher G, Frisch H, Pollak A: Pulsatile secretion of gonadotrophins in early infancy. Eur J Pediatr 137:71–74, 1981.

7. Conte FA, Grumbach MM, Kaplan SL: A diphasic pattern of gonadotrophin secretion in patients with the syndrome of gonadal dysegenesis. J Clin Endocrinol Metab 40:670–675, 1975.

8. Conte FA, Grumbach MM, Kaplan SL, Reiter EO: Correlation of LRF induced LH and FSH release from infancy to 19 years with the changing pattern of gonadotrophin secretion in agonadal patients: Relation to the restraint of puberty. J Clin Endocrinol Metab 50:163–168, 1980.

9. Noonan JJ, Nass TE, Terasawa E: Lesions of the posterior hypothalamus induce precocious puberty in female rhesus monkeys (Abstract Number 125). The Endocrine Society, 62nd Annual Meeting, pp 106, 1980.

10. Tanner JM: A history of the study of human growth. Cambridge: Cambridge University Press, 1981, pp 286–298.

11. Zacharias L, Wurtman RJ: Age at menarche, genetic and environmental influences. N Engl J Med 280:868–875, 1969.

12. Reiter RR: The pineal gland and its hormones in the control of reproduction in mammals. Endocrinol Rev 1:109–131, 1980.

13. Silman RE, Leone RM, Hooper RJL, Preece MA: Melatonin, the pineal gland and human puberty. Nature 282:301–303, 1979.

14. Lenko HL, Lang U, Aubert ML, Paunier L, Sizonenko PO: Hormonal changes in puberty. VII. Lack of variation of daytime plasma melatonin. J Clin Endocrinol Metab 54:1056–1058, 1982.

15. Sklar CA, Conte FA, Kaplan SL, Grumbach MM: Human chorionic gonadotrophin-secreting pineal tumour: Relation to pathogenesis and sex limitation of sexual precocity. J Clin Endocrinol Metab 53:656–660, 1981.

16. Grumbach MM, Richards GE, Conte FA, Kaplan SL: Clinical disorders of adrenal function and puberty: An assessment of the role of the adrenal cortex in normal and abnormal puberty in man and evidence for an ACTH-like pituitary adrenal androgen stimulating hormone. In James VHT, Serio M, Giusti G, Martini L (eds): The Endocrine Function of the Human Adrenal Cortex. London, New York, San Francisco: Academic Press, pp 583–612, 1978.

17. Silverman SH, Migeon C, Rosenberg E, Wilkins L: Precocious growth of sexual hair without other secondary sexual development, "premature pubarche." A constitutional variation of adolescence. Pediatrician 10:426–431, 1952.

18. Boyar R, Finkelstein J, Roffwarg H, Kapen S, Weitzman E, Hellman L: Synchronization of augmented LH secretion with sleep during puberty; N Engl J Med 287:582–586, 1972.

19. Wu FCW, Butler GE, Kelnar CJH, Sellar RE: Patterns of pulsatile luteinizing hormone secretion before and during the onset of puberty in boys: A study using an immunoradiometric assay. J Clin Endocrinol Metab 70:629–637, 1990.

20. Penny R, Olambiwonnu NO, Frasier SD: Episodic fluctuation of serum gonadotrophins in pre- and post-pubertal boys and girls. J Clin Endocrinol Metab 45:307–311, 1977.

21. Crowley WF, Comite F, Vale WW, Rivier J, Loriaux DL, Cutler GB: Therapeutic use of pituitary desensitization with a long acting LH-RH agonist: A potential new treatment for idiopathic precocious puberty. J Clin Endocrinol Metab 52:370–372, 1981.

22. Shalet SM: Gonadal function following radiation and cytotoxic chemotherapy in childhood. Ergebnisse der Inneren Medizin und Kinderheilkunde, Bd 58, Springer-Verlang, Berlin, Heidelberg, 1989.

23. Whitehead E, Shalet SM, Morris-Jones PH, Beardwell CG, Deakin DP: Gonadal function after combination chemotherapy for Hodgkin's disease in childhood. Arch Dis Child 57:287–291, 1982.

24. Clayton PE, Shalet SM, Price DA, Campbell RHA: Testicular damage after chemotherapy for childhood brain tumors. J Pediatr 112:922–926, 1989.

25. Clayton PE, Shalet SM, Price DA, Morris-Jones PH: Ovarian function following chemotherapy for childhood brain tumors. Med Pediatr Oncol 17:92–96, 1989.

26. Dunkel L, Alfthan H, Stenman UH, Perheentupa J: Gonadal control of pulsatile secretion of lutenizing hormone and follicle stimulating hormone in prepubertal boys evaluated by ultrasensitive time-resolved immunofluormetric assays. J Clin Endocrinol Metab 70:104–107, 1990.

12

Precocious and Premature Puberty Following Prophylactic Cranial Irradiation in Acute Lymphoblastic Leukemia

R. Stanhope, M.D., A. Papadimitriou, M.D., J. M. Chessells, M.D., and A. D. Leiper, M.B.

Cranial irradiation (CRT) causes pituitary dysfunction when given in high doses for the treatment of tumors of the central nervous system (CNS) that are distant from the hypothalamo-pituitary region. Growth hormone (GH) deficiency [1], delayed puberty [2,3], and precocious puberty [4,5] have been described. Initial reports of precocious puberty as a consequence of CRT were associated with high doses of CRT used in the treatment of solid brain tumors [5]. The prognosis for children with acute lymphoblastic leukemia (ALL) improved dramatically with the introduction of prophylactic treatment for prevention of leukemic infiltration of the CNS. Such prophylaxis commonly comprises a combination of fractionated low-dose CRT (1,800–2,400 cGy) combined with a course of intrathecal methotrexate (IT MTX). Certainly, CNS prophylactic regimens can cause combinations of GH deficiency/insufficiency [1,6,7] and premature/precocious puberty [8,9]. Most children receiving CNS prophylaxis with CRT probably do not require GH supplements [10]. The combination of GH insufficiency and premature/precocious puberty may be associated with a compromised [9] or absent [11] pubertal growth spurt and result in severe growth failure. Such children should be identified at an early stage and assessed for endocrine therapy. We have treated eight girls with premature/precocious puberty resulting from CNS prophylaxis for ALL with either a gonadotrophin releasing hormone (GnRH) analog or a combination of GnRH analog and biosynthetic GH. We report the effects on growth rate and growth prognosis after 2.5 years of treatment.

PATIENTS AND METHODS

Our patient group has previously been described [11]. Between 1971 and 1988, 788 children were referred for ALL, of which 514 were alive in January 1988. Two hundred and fifty-five patients were more than 6.5 years of age and had been treated with CRT at less than eight years of age. They had not received gonadal irradiation. All were treated by standard protocols [12–14], which included IT MTX. From 1972, prophylactic CRT of 2,400 cGy was given in 15 fractions over 19 days. This was reduced to 1,800 cGy in 10 fractions over 12 days in January 1981.

Eight girls with precocious or premature puberty were treated for abnormal growth. The clinical details are given in Table 1. The mean age for the onset of puberty was 7.90 years (6.8–10.1) and all

Late Effects of Treatment for Childhood Cancer, pages 89–94 © 1992 Wiley-Liss, Inc.

TABLE 1. Clinical Data of Eight Girls Treated for Acute Lymphoblastic
Leukemia With Precocious or Premature Onset of Puberty

Patient	Age at diagnosis (years)	CRT (cGy)	Age at onset of puberty (years)	Treatment
1	4.6	1800	8.3	GnRHa + GH
2	4.5	1800	8.1	GnRHa + GH
3	4.3	1800	6.8	GnRHa + GH
4	3.1	1800	7.0	GnRHa + GH
5	3.4	1800	7.5	GnRHa + GH
6	2.4	1800	7.1	GnRHa + GH
7	6.8	1800	10.1	GnRHa
8	1.8	2400	8.0	GnRHa
Mean range	3.9		7.9	
	(1.8–6.8)		(6.8–10.1)	

GH = growth hormone; GnRHa = gonadotrophin releasing hormone analog; CRT =
cranial irradiation.

had an absent growth spurt of puberty.
Growth was assessed at three monthly intervals using standard anthropometric
techniques [15]. Epiphysial maturation
was assessed by one observer (RS) using
the method of Tanner et al. [16]. Growth
hormone secretion was measured in response to insulin-induced hypoglycemia
by standard techniques [17].

The GnRH analog therapy was administered as a depot preparation of (D-Ser 6)
GnRH as a monthly injection of 3.6 mg of
goserelin (Zoladex). Natural sequence biosynthetic human GH was administered in
a dose regimen of 15–20 U/m²/week as a
daily subcutaneous injection given during
the evening. Statistical analysis was paired
student's *t*-test.

RESULTS

The group of 255 patients comprised
121 girls and 134 boys. The onset of puberty at less than two standard deviations
(SD) of the mean occurred in 24 girls
(20%), which was more than would have
been expected from the normal distribution (3%). Four boys (3%) entered puberty
at less than two SD from the mean, which
was compatible with the normal distribution. Seven girls and two boys had precocious puberty. Growth data from five
girls with absent growth spurts are shown
in Fig. 1. The combination of an absent
growth spurt at puberty associated with
premature or precocious puberty may result in severe growth failure.

Growth hormone insufficiency (peak
GH to hypoglycemia <20 m U/L) was
demonstrated in six of the eight patients,
whereas the other two had peak GH levels
just above 20 m U/L. There are no normal
values for pharmacological tests of GH secretion during the growth spurt of girls
with premature sexual maturation. It is
probable that even the highest GH level
attained in the eight girls (23 m U/L) was
an indication of GH insufficiency.

The results of treatment with GnRH analog alone in patients seven and eight are
shown in Fig. 2. The GnRH analog treatment was associated with a slowing in the
rate of epiphysial maturation (Fig. 3a), but
there was, nonetheless, a dramatic growth
deceleration that persisted during treatment. The resulting height prognosis

(height SDS for bone age) showed no significant alteration (Fig. 2). Six girls were treated with a combination of GnRH analog and biosynthetic human GH. The former permitted slowing of the rate of epiphysial maturation, while the latter allowed a growth acceleration (Fig. 3b). During 2.5 years of combined treatment, the mean height SDS for bone age increased from +0.61 to +0.92 ($P<0.05$) (Fig. 4). Five patients showed a gradual increase in height SDS for bone age with treatment, but one showed no alteration.

DISCUSSION

Our data suggest that premature and precocious puberty are sequelae of CNS prophylaxis for ALL. This occurred irre-

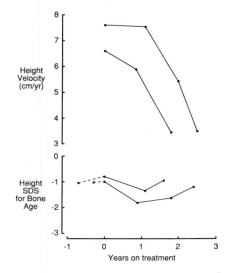

Fig. 2. Height velocity and height SDS for bone age data from patients 7 and 8 treated with GnRH analog alone. The dotted lines represent pretreatment data.

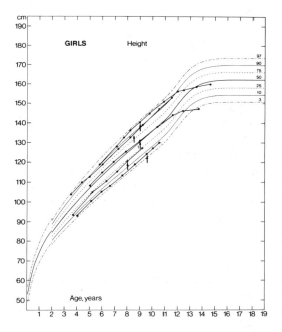

Fig. 1. Growth data from five girls treated for ALL, including low-dose CRT and IT MTX for CNS prophylaxis, who had no growth acceleration at the onset of breast development. None had received spinal irradiation. The onset of breast stage 2 is indicated by the vertical arrows [11].

spective of whether the irradiation dose was 1,800 or 2,400 cGy and the role of IT MTX could not be differentiated from CRT. Precocious and premature puberty in untreated children was much more common in girls than boys. This is the same sex distribution as occurs in idiopathic central precocious puberty [18], and indeed, the mean age of the onset of puberty is earlier in normal girls than boys [19]. Constitutional delay of puberty is more common in boys [18]. This interesting sex distribution for the onset of puberty is reflected in treatment regimens. It is easier to induce puberty in girls with delayed puberty using pulsatile GnRH therapy [20]; in contrast, it is more difficult to suppress central precocious puberty in girls using a GnRH analog [21]. We suggest that the growth of girls who have had CNS prophylaxis for ALL, especially if treated at an early age, should be closely monitored and that signs of secondary sexual characteristics observed and related to their rate of growth.

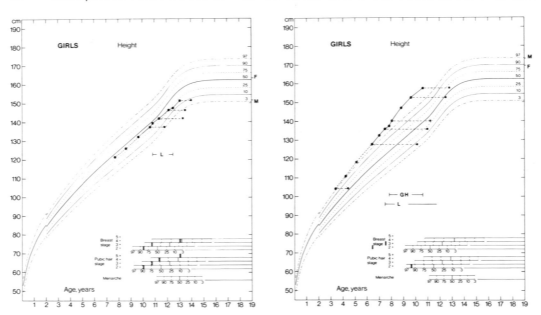

Fig. 3. Growth data from patient 7 (left) and patient 5 (right). Patient 7 was treated with GnRH analog alone, whereas patient 5 was treated with a combination of GnRH analog (L) and growth hormone (GH). Epiphysial maturation is shown as solid squares and the parental centiles [Maternal (M) and paternal (F)] are shown on the right-hand border.

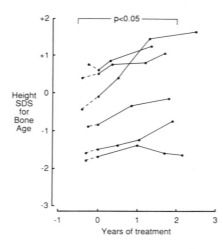

Fig. 4. Height SDS for bone age data from 6 girls treated with a combination of GnRH analog and GH. Pretreatment data are shown as broken lines.

The intensity of the growth spurt of puberty is dependent on chronological age [22]. Children with precocious puberty should attain a peak height velocity of a much greater magnitude than normal children entering puberty within the normal range. The absence or impairment of this spontaneous growth spurt in girls treated with low-dose CRT and IT MTX may lead to severe growth impairment. This occurs as epiphysial maturation proceeds at a rapid rate producing epiphysial closure without an associated increase in linear growth. The use of a GnRH analog suppresses signs of sexual maturation and slows the rate of epiphysial maturation, but there is also a marked growth deceleration [23,24]. In children who already have GH insufficiency and are growing at a less than optimum rate, such a growth deceleration associated with GnRH analog treatment would be detrimental. In idiopathic central precocious puberty, it is highly probable that GnRH analogs do not improve final height prognosis [25]. We have adopted a combined regimen for this reason, and used GH treatment to sustain or increase growth rate, while a GnRH analog was administered to reduce the rate of epiphysial maturation. Although our results only extend to a period of 2.5 years, there is a suggestion that final height prognosis is increased by this joint regimen. Height prognosis in untreated central precocious puberty can, however, be difficult to interpret, and may show an increase when observed over short periods of time [26]. Longer treatment periods will be required to assess the effect of the combined regimen of GnRH analog and GH treatment on final height.

REFERENCES

1. Shalet SM: Irradiation-induced growth failure. Clin Endocrinol Metab 15:591–606, 1986.
2. Styne DM, Grumbach MM: Puberty in the male and female: Its physiology and disorders. In Yen SSC, Jaff RB (eds): Reproductive Endocrinology. Philadelphia: WB Saunders, 1976, pp 189–240.
3. Rappaport R, Brauner R, Czernichow P et al.: Effect of hypothalamic and pituitary irradiation on pubertal development in children with cranial tumors. J Clin Endocrinol Metab 54:1164–1168, 1982.
4. Brauner R, Czernichow P, Reppaport R: Precocious puberty after hypothalamic and pituitary irradiation in young children. N Engl J Med 311:920, 1984.
5. Brauner R, Rappaport R: Precocious puberty secondary to cranial irradiation for tumors distant from the hypothalamopituitary area. Horm Res 22:78–82, 1985.
6. Shalet SM, Beardwell CG, Twomey JA, Morris-Jones PH, Pearson D: Endocrine function following the treatment of acute leukemia in childhood. J Pediatr 90:920–923, 1977.
7. Kirk JA, Raghupathy P, Steens MM et al.: Growth failure and growth hormone deficiency after treatment for acute lymphoblastic leukemia. Lancet i:190–193, 1987.
8. Moell C, Garwicz S, Westgren U, Wiebe T: Disturbed pubertal growth in girls treated for acute lymphoblastic leukemia. Pediatr Hem Oncol 4:1–5, 1987.
9. Leiper AD, Stanhope R, Kitching P, Chessells JM: Precocious and premature puberty associated with treatment of acute lymphoblastic leukemia. Arch Dis Child 62:1107–1112, 1987.
10. Robison LL, Nesbit ME, Sather HN, Meadows AT, Ortega JA, Hammond GD: Height of children successfully treated for acute lymphoblastic leukemia: A report from the late effects study committee of children's cancer study group. Med Pediatr Oncol 13:14–21, 1985.
11. Leiper AD, Stanhope R, Preece MA, Grant DB, Chessells JM: Precocious or early puberty and growth failure in girls treated for acute lymphoblastic leukemia. Horm Res 30:72–76, 1988.
12. Chessells JM, Ninane J, Tiedemann K: Present problems in management of childhood lymphoblastic leukemia. Experience from the Hospital for Sick Children, London. In Neth R, Gallo RC, Graaf T, Mannweiler R (eds): Modern Trends in Human Leukemia. Berlin: Springer-Verlag, 1981, pp 108–114.
13. Chessells JM, Leiper AD, Tiedemann K et al.: Oral methotrexate is as effective as intramuscular methotrexate in maintenance therapy of acute lymphoblastic leukemia. Arch Dis Child 62:172–176, 1987.
14. Pinkerton CR, Bowman A, Holzel H, Chessells JM: Intensive consolidation chemotherapy for acute lymphoblastic leukemia. Arch Dis Child 62:12–18, 1987.
15. Brook CGD (ed): Growth Assessment in Childhood and Adolescence. Oxford: Blackwell Press, 1982.
16. Tanner JM, Whitehouse RH, Cameron N et al. (eds): Assessment of Skeletal Maturity and Prediction of Adult Height (TW2 method). London: Academic Press, 1983.
17. Hughes IA (ed): Handbook of Endocrine Tests in Children. Bristol: Wright, 1986.
18. Stanhope R, Brook CGD: Disorders of puberty. In Brook CGD (ed): Clinical Paediatric Endocrinology. 2nd ed. Oxford: Blackwell Press, 1989 pp 189–212.
19. Brook CGD, Stanhope R: Normal puberty: Physical characteristics and endocrinology. In Brook CGD (ed): Clinical Paediatric Endocrinology. 2nd ed. Oxford: Blackwell Press. 1989, pp 169–188.
20. Stanhope R, Brook CGD, Pringle PJ, Adams J,

Jacobs HS: Induction of puberty by pulsatile gonadotrophin releasing hormone. Lancet ii: 552–555, 1987.

21. Donaldson MDC, Stanhope R, Lee TJ et al.: Gonadoprophin responses to GnRH in precocious puberty treated with GnRH analogue. Clin Endocrinol 21:499–503, 1984.

22. Tanner JM (ed): Foetus into man. London: Open Books, 1986.

23. Luder AS, Holland FJ, Costigan DC et al.: Intranasal and subcutaneous treatment of central precocious puberty in both sexes with a long-acting analogue of luteinizing hormone-releasing hormone. J Clin Endocrinol Metab 58:966–972, 1984.

24. Mansfield MJ, Beardsworth DE, Loughlin JS et al.: Long-term treatment of central precocious puberty with a long-acting analogue of luteinizing hormone-releasing hormone: Effects on somatic growth and skeletal maturation. N Engl J Med 309:1286–1290, 1983.

25. Stanhope R, Pringle PJ, Grook CGD: Growth hormone and sex steroid secretion in girls with central precocious puberty treated with GnRH analogue. Acta Pediatr Scand 77:525–530, 1988.

26. Werder EA, Murset G, Zachmann M, Brook CGD, Prader A: Treatment of precocious puberty with cyproterone acetate. Pediatr Res 8:248–256, 1974.

13

Effects of Bone Marrow Transplantation on Reproductive Function

Jean E. Sanders, M.D., and the Seattle Marrow Transplant Team

As the success of marrow transplantation has steadily improved over the past two decades, the number of patients receiving this procedure has increased, which, in turn, has resulted in an increasing number of long-term survivors [1]. Marrow transplantation is now the treatment of choice for young patients with severe aplastic anemia who have suitably matched donors, and represents the only possible cure for patients with some inherited disorders [2–5]. Compared with other types of treatment, marrow transplantation offers an improved disease-free survival advantage for selected patients with a variety of hematologic malignancies [6–9]. An important factor that results in additional patients being able to receive marrow transplants is the expansion of the marrow donor pool to include related and unrelated individuals who are partially or fully HLA matched with the patient [10–12].

Marrow transplant preparative regimens usually utilize high-dose alkylating agent therapy either alone or in combination with total body irradiation (TBI). Chemotherapy and irradiation induced damage to the mature gonad with resultant sterility has been observed among patients who receive conventional chemotherapy and/or localized radiation therapy [13,14]. Treatment of children and adolescents with chemotherapy and/or radiation therapy may influence the ability of these children subsequently to progress normally through puberty and achieve normal reproductive function [14]. Since most marrow transplant patients are children or young adults, the potential injury of the transplant preparative regimen to the reproductive system is of concern. This chapter discusses the late effects of gonadal function that have been described to date among long-term survivors after marrow transplantation.

CHEMOTHERAPY PREPARATIVE REGIMENS

Prior to marrow transplantation most patients with severe aplastic anemia receive cyclophosphamide (CY) given as a single agent in divided doses up to 200 mg/kg to suppress the immune system [2,3]. Patients with nonmalignant hematologic disorders, such as thalassemia major or Wiscott Aldrich syndrome, receive additional marrow ablation with 14–16 mg/kg-total doses of busulfan (BU) in addition to the high doses of CY [4,5]. This same regimen of high-dose BU + CY is also given to patients with hematologic malignancies [15]. Alkylating agents have been associated with gonadal damage that may result in teratogenesis and transient or persistent infertility. The patient's age at time of treatment, total drug dose administered, and the duration of therapy, as well as patient sex and sexual maturity, are variables that have been important predictors of damage to the gonad [14,16].

Women

Women who have been treated with alkylating agents may have significant impairment of reproductive function. Among women who received CY therapy, ova and thecal cell loss on ovarian biopsies suggests a direct action of the drug on the oocyte [17]. The potential reversibility of this loss has been found to be related to the total dose of CY given and patient age. Women over 40 years of age who received a total dose of 5.0g CY developed amenorrhea, but women 20–30 years of age required a total dose of 20.0 g to result in amenorrhea [13,17]. Thus, the ovarian function and fertility of older women given high-dose CY is more likely to be compromised.

Following 200 mg/kg CY and marrow transplantation for aplastic anemia, ovarian function has been evaluated in 51 women who were postpubertal at the time of the marrow transplant [18–25]. All 33 patients who were between the ages of 13 and 25 years recovered ovarian function. This occurred between three and 42 months after CY administration and marrow transplant and was documented with normal gonadotropin levels and return of regular menstrual cycles. Ten of 18 women who were between 26 and 38 years of transplant had evidence of ovarian function recovery. Eight women never had return of normal ovarian function and four of the 10 who recovered have subsequently developed ovarian failure. These 12 women have primary ovarian failure with elevated gonadotropin levels, low estradiol levels, and amenorrhea. Increasing patient age was the only factor significantly associated with ovarian function abnormalities following 200 mg/kg CY [19].

Very little information is available for women who received high-dose BU + CY for marrow transplant preparation. Two patients transplanted for thalassemia and 10 patients transplanted for hematologic malignancies have had gonadal function evaluations performed [26]. All have low levels of estradiol (>20 pg/ml) and elevated levels of luteinizing hormone (LH) and follicle stimulating hormone (FSH).

Girls

The prepubertal gonad may be more resistant to alkylating agent therapy than the postpubertal gonad, but primary ovarian failure may occur in girls given CY before puberty [13,27]. It has been estimated that less than 10% of girls who receive CY develop elevated FSH levels and morphologic changes consistent with impaired follicle maturation. Doses of >500 mg/kg of CY are needed before ovarian abnormalities have been observed in young girls. Following 200 mg/kg CY and marrow transplantation for aplastic anemia, 23 prepubertal girls who were between the ages of two and 12 years at the time of transplant have been evaluated at a median of nine years after transplant [28]. Eighteen of these 23 are now more than 12 years of age and 17 have developed normally through puberty. These 17 girls have normal LH and FSH levels, as well as normal estradiol and regular menustration. Menarche occurred at a median of 12 years of age. No data are yet available regarding pubertal development and hormone function in prepubertal girls who received high-dose BU and CY.

Men

The predominant lesion demonstrated in the adult male given alkylating agent therapy is localized to the germinal epithelium of the testes [13]. Testicular biopsies demonstrate that these men may develop germinal aplasia, absent spermatogonia, and spermatozoa but have normal appearing Leydig cells [29,30]. They have elevated FSH levels and azoospermia with normal LH and testosterone levels. The total dose of CY received appears to be important for men. Those who receive 4.5 mg/kg/day of CY for less than two months retain normal gonadal function; treatment for more than three months may result in oliogospermia and total doses of 18 g usually result in azoospermia [30,31]. After a period of time following discontinuation of the drug, recovery of spermatogenesis has been observed.

Testicular function has been evaluated one year or more after 200 mg/kg CY and marrow transplantation for aplastic anemia in 55 postpubertal men [18,32]. All had normal testosterone levels and 53 had normal LH levels. FSH values were elevated in 21 patients. Semen analysis, when tested, was normal for 66% of the men and demonstrated azoospermia for the remainder.

Little information is available for males who received the high-dose BU + CY preparative regimen for hematologic malignancy. Four patients have been evaluated one year after marrow transplant. They demonstrated normal LH and testosterone levels and minimally elevated FSH levels. Semen analysis performed on two patients demonstrated sperm.

Boys

The germinal epithelium of the prepubertal testes is susceptible to damage induced by CY. Testicular biopsies have demonstrated aplasia of the germinal epithelium. These patients also have high serum FSH levels [33]. A dose of >360 mg/kg seems to be required before damage is observed in prepubertal or pubertal boys.

After 200 mg/kg CY and marrow transplantation for aplastic anemia, 18 prepubertal boys who were 2–13 years of age at the time of transplant have been evaluated at a median of nine years after transplant [28]. All boys who are now more than 13 years of age have shown normal progression through puberty with Tanner developmental scores appropriate for their chronological age. The LH, FSH, and testosterone levels are also normal. Eight of these boys have had semen analysis performed. Two demonstrated azoospermia and six had normal sperm counts.

More data are needed before definitive statements can be made regarding gonadal function after BU + CY preparative regimen among prepubertal boys. To date, only seven boys have been studied [26]. At one year, three demonstrated normal gonadatropin levels and testosterone values were normal. Four boys, however, have abnormal FSH and LH levels after stimulation with gonadatropin releasing hormone but low testosterone levels. These four boys have delayed development.

Fertility

Cytotoxic therapy given to men prior to or at the time of conception usually does not result in congenital abnormalities in children fathered by these men [34]. Chemotherapy administered to women just prior to conception or after the first trimester usually does not jeopardize the unborn child [35,36]. Patients who have been treated with chemotherapy may have increased fetal wastage, however. A total of 55 children are known to have been born to 36 patients who received marrow transplant preparative regimens consisting of chemotherapy only (Table 1) [18–25].

PREPARATIVE REGIMENS CONTAINING TOTAL BODY IRRADIATION

The marrow transplant preparative regimen for most patients with hematologic

TABLE 1. Fertility After Marrow Transplantation[a]

Preparative regimen	Cyclophosphamide		Cyclophosphamide + total body irradiation	
Patient sex	Women	Men	Women	Men
Number of patients	15	21	4	2
Number of pregnancies	25	28	5	4
Number of abortions	4	0	4	0
Number of live births	21	28	1	4

[a]From [18–25, 48, 49].

malignancies includes TBI [6–12]. Total doses of 7.5–10.0 Gy have been given as a single exposure or total doses of 12.0–15.75 Gy have been administered over 4–7 days. Dose rates range from 5 to 26 cGy/min. In addition, most of the TBI regimens include chemotherapy with CY or other cytotoxic agents. Some preparative regimens for patients with nonmalignant hematologic disorders also include TBI given in lower doses of 2.0–3.0 Gy or total lymphoid irradiation [37]. Ionizing irradiation is known to have an adverse effect on gonadal function of all patients and the ability to recover from these effects appears to be related to the dose given and the patient age at the time of irradiation [14].

Women

Age and total dose of irradiation received by the adult ovary are factors determining ovarian failure. Women older than 40 years require doses of only 6.0 Gy to result in permanent ovarian failure, whereas up to 50% of the younger women will recover gonadal function with doses up to 20.0 Gy [14,38].

After transplant of preparative regimens containing TBI or total lymphoid irradiation, 160 postpubertal women have been evaluated at one or more years after transplant [18,19,28,29,39,40]. All 60 women treated with single fraction TBI had primary ovarian failure with elevated LH and FSH levels, low estradiol levels, and amenorrhea. Two women who were less than 25 years of age had recovery of ovarian function with normalization of gonadotropins and estradiol, as well as return of spontaneous menstruation 5–6 years after transplant. The remaining 100 women all received fractionated TBI with total doses of 12.0–15.75 Gy. They all developed primary ovarian failure for at least three years. Seven who were less than 25 years of age have had return of ovarian function after 3–4 years.

Girls

There are no studies that directly address the late effects of irradiation on the prepubertal ovary. After TBI and marrow transplantation, 27 girls who were prepubertal at the time are now beyond 12 years of age and evaluable for pubertal development [28,39,41]. Development of secondary sexual characteristics was delayed for 14 and normal for 13. These 13 girls achieved menarche by a median of 13 years of age (11–15). Gonadotropin levels were normal for those who developed normally, and were elevated for those girls with delayed development who have benefited from appropriate hormone supplementation.

Men

Studies of the irradiated adult testes have demonstrated that the magnitude and duration of suppression of spermatogenesis are dependent on the dose [14]. Doses as low as 0.3 Gy result in germinal epithelial damage, decreased sperm counts and increased FSH levels [42].

Leydig cell function is usually spared and testosterone levels are normal. Return of sperm counts and FSH values to preirradiation levels after single exposure radiation doses of 3.0 Gy may occur after 30 months; after higher doses, up to five years are needed before recovery has been observed. No patient has been documented to have recovery of testicular function after fractionated doses of irradiation [43].

Testicular function has been evaluated in 170 men after TBI for marrow transplantation [18,28,32,39,41]. Testosterone levels were normal, LH levels were slightly elevated in 22%, and FSH were elevated in 77%. Semen analysis demonstrated azoospermia in all men up to seven years after transplant. Two men who received single exposure TBI had recovery of spermatogenesis between seven and eight years thereafter.

Boys

Irradiation to the prepubertal testes results in damage to the testicular germinal epithelium that does not become apparent until after puberty [44]. Boys given 24-Gy testicular irradiation have delayed sexual maturation, elevated gonadotropin levels, and low testosterone levels [45,46]. Among 45 boys who were prepubertal at time of marrow transplant and are now evaluable for pubertal development, delayed development occurred in 27 [28,29,41]. All 11 of the boys who received testicular irradiation of 18.0–24.0 Gy in addition to TBI have delayed development and gonadal failure with elevated FSH and LH levels and testosterone levels >100 ng/dL. These boys required hormore supplementation to develop secondary sexual characteristics. Those who received only TBI had variable LH and FSH levels, but the majority had normal LH levels with elevated FSH levels. Testosterone levels were normal among the boys with normal development and low among the delayed development.

Fertility

Irradiation of germ cells may induce mutations that could result in congenital abnormalities in the progeny of those treated patients who recover gonadal function. The risk of serious hereditary abnormalities within the first two generations after irradiation of either parent has been estimated to be approximately 100 cases/million/Gray of exposure [47]. Thus a patient exposed to 10.0–15.75 Gy TBI would have about 10–15% of germ cells affected. Some clinical studies have shown no increase in abnormalities of offspring or of spontaneous abortions of individuals exposed to irradiation.

A total of 12 pregnancies are known to have occurred following TBI containing marrow transplant preparative regimens [18,19,48,49]. Eight of these occurred in seven women between three and eight years after transplant. Three pregnancies have resulted in the birth of a normal baby, one woman is still pregnant, and four have resulted in spontaneous abortions. Two men have been known to father four children, all of which are normal.

SUMMARY

Both normal and abnormal reproductive function has been observed following marrow transplantation. Important factors in predicting this include the age and sex of the patient and the type of transplant preparative regimen received. Children who receive CY only preparative regimens appear to develop through puberty normally and have normal gonadal function. There is not enough data yet available to know the impact of high-dose BU + CY on pubertal development. Development may be delayed after TBI, however. Women less than 25 years of age who received CY only regimens appear to have normal gonadal function recovery as do some of the older women. Similarly, men given only CY usually have normal testicular function. Primary ovarian failure is most likely to occur following TBI containing regimens and most men are infertile. These factors should be considered when counseling patients prior to marrow transplantation.

ACKNOWLEDGMENTS

This investigation was supported by Grant Number HL 36444 awarded by the National Heart, Lung and Blood Institute and Grant Numbers CA 18029, CA 26828, CA 18221, CA 09515, and CA 15704 awarded by the National Cancer Institute.

REFERENCES

1. Bortin MM, Rimm AA: Increasing utilization of bone marrow transplantation. Transplantation 42:229–234, 1986.

2. Sanders JE, Whitehead J, Storb R, et al.: Bone marrow transplantation experience for children with aplastic anemia. Pediatr 77:179–186, 1986.

3. Storb R, Deeg HJ, Pepe M, et al.: Methotrexate and cyclosporine versus cyclosporine alone for prophyalaxis of graft-versus-host disease in patients given HLA-identical marrow grafts for leukemia: Long-term follow-up of a controlled trial. Blood 73:1729–1734, 1989.

4. Lucarelli G, Galimberti M, Polchi P, et al.: Bone marrow transplantation in patients with thalassemia. N Engl J Med 322:417–421, 1990.

5. O'Reilly RJ, Brochstein J, Dinsmore JR, Kirkpatrick D: Marrow transplantation for congenital disorders. Sem Hematol 21:188–221, 1984.

6. Woods WG, Nesbit ME, Ramsay NKC, et al.: Intensive therapy followed by bone marrow transplantation for patients with acute lymphocytic leukemia in second or subsequent remission: Determination of prognostic factors (A report from the University of Minnesota Bone Marrow Transplantation Team). Blood 61:1182–1189, 1983.

7. Thomas ED, Clift RA, Fefer A, et al.: Marrow transplantation for the treatment of chronic myelogenous leukemia. Ann Intern Med 104:155–163, 1986.

8. Clift RA, Buckner CD, Thomas ED, et al.: The treatment of acute non-lymphoblastic leukemia by allogeneic marrow transplantation. Bone Marrow Transplantation 2:243–258, 1987.

9. Appelbaum FR, Barrall J, Storb R, et al.: Bone marrow transplantation for patients with myelodysplasia. Pretreatment variables and outcome. Ann Inter Med 112:590–597, 1990.

10. Beatty PG, Clift RA, Mickelson EM, et al.: Marrow transplantation from related donors other than HLA-identical siblings. N Engl J Med 313:765–771, 1985.

11. Beatty PG, Hansen JA, Longton GM, et al.: Marrow transplantation from HLA-matched unrelated donors for treatment of hematologic malignancies. Transplantation 51:443–447, 1991.

12. Ash RC, Casper JT, Chitambar CR, et al.: Successful allogeneic transplantation of T-cell-depleted bone marrow from closely HLA-matched unrelated donors. N Engl J Med 322:485–494, 1990.

13. Shalet SM: Effects of cancer chemotherapy on gonadal function of patients. Cancer Treat Rev 7:131–152, 1980.

14. Kay H, Mattison D: How radiation and chemotherapy affect gonadal function. Contemp Ob Gyn 109:106–115, 1985.

15. Santos GW, Tutschka PJ, Brookmeyer R, et al.: Marrow transplantation for acute non-lymphocytic leukemia after treatment with busulfan and cyclophosphamide. N Engl J Med 309:1347–1353, 1983.

16. Chapman RM: Effect of cytotoxic therapy on sexuality and gonadal function. Semin Oncol 9:84–92, 1982.

17. Warne GL, Fairley KF, Hobbs JB, Martin FIR: Cyclophosphamide-induced ovarian failure. N Engl J Med 289:1159–1162, 1973.

18. Sanders JE, Buckner CD, Leonard JM, et al.: Late effects on gonadal function of cyclophosphamide, total-body irradiation, and marrow transplantation. Transplantation 36: 252–255, 1983.

19. Sanders JE, Buckner CD, Amos D, et al.: Ovarian function following marrow transplantation for aplastic anemia or leukemia. J Clin Oncol 6:813–818, 1988.

20. Hinterberger-Fischer M, Hinterberger W, Hayek-Rosenmayr A, et al.: Pregnancy and delivery after bone marrow transplantation for severe aplastic anemia. Blut 54:313–315, 1987.

21. Milliken S, Powles R, Parikh P, et al.: Successful pregnancy following bone marrow transplantation for leukemia. Bone Marrow Transplantation 5:135–137, 1990.

22. Card RT, Holmes IH, Sugarman RG, Storb R, Thomas ED: Successful pregnancy after high dose chemotherapy and marrow transplantation for treatment of aplastic anemia. Exp Hematol 8:57–60, 1980.

23. Jacobs P, Dubovsky DW: Bone marrow trans-

plantation followed by normal pregnancy. Am J Hematol 11:209–212, 1981.

24. Deeg HJ, Kennedy MS, Sanders JE, Thomas ED, Storb R: Successful pregnancy after marrow transplantation for severe aplastic anemia and immunosuppression with cyclosporine. JAMA 250:647, 1983.

25. Schmidt H, Ehninger G, Dopfer R, Waller HD: Pregnancy after bone marrow transplantation for severe aplastic anemia. Bone Marrow Transplantation 2:329–332, 1987.

26. Manenti F, Galimberti M, Lucarelli G, et al.: Growth and endocrine function after bone marrow transplantation for thalassemia. In Buckner CD, Gale RP and Lucarelli G (eds): Advances and Controversies in Thalassemia Therapy: Bone Marrow Transplantation and Other Approaches. New York: Alan R. Liss, 1989, pp 273–280.

27. Nicosia SV, Matus-Ridley M, Meadows AT: Gonadal effects of cancer therapy in girls. Cancer 55:2364–2372, 1985.

28. Sanders JE, Buckner CD, Sullivan KM, et al.: Growth and development in children after bone marrow transplantation. Horm Res 30:92–97, 1988.

29. Fairley KF, Barrie JU, Johnson W: Sterility and testicular atrophy related to cyclophosphamide therapy. Lancet 1:568–569, 1972.

30. Etteldorf JN, West CD, Pitcock JA, Williams DL: Gonadal function, testicular histology, and meiosis following cyclophosphamide therapy in patients with nephrotic syndrome. J Pediatr 88:206–212, 1976.

31. Buchanan JD, Fairley KF, Barrie JU: Return of spermatogenesis after stopping cyclophosphamide therapy. Lancet 2:156–157, 1975.

32. Sklar CA, Kim TH, Ramsay NKC: Testicular function following bone marrow transplantation performed during or after puberty. Cancer 53:1498–1501, 1984.

33. Lentz RD, Bergstein J, Steffes MW, et al.: Postpubertal evaluation of gonadal function following cyclophosphamide therapy before and during puberty. J Pediatr 91:385–394, 1977.

34. Holmes GF, Holmes FF: Pregnancy outcome of patients treated for Hodgkin's disease. Cancer 41:1317–1322, 1978.

35. Li FP, Fine W, Jaffe N, Holmes G, Holmes F: Offspring of patients treated for cancer in childhood. J Natl Cancer Inst 62:1193–1197, 1979.

36. Blatt J, Mulvihill JJ, Ziegler JL, Young RC, Poplack DG: Pregnancy outcome following cancer chemotherapy. Am J Med 69:828–832, 1980.

37. Ramsay NKC, Kim T, Nesbit ME, et al.: Total lymphoid irradiation and cyclophosphamide as preparation for bone marrow transplantation for severe aplastic anemia. Blood 55:344–346, 1980.

38. Lushbaugh CC, Caserett GW: The effects of gonadal irradiation in clinical radiation therapy. A review. Cancer 37:1111–1120, 1976.

39. Sanders JE, Pritchard S, Mahoney P, et al.: Growth and development following marrow transplantation for leukemia. Blood 68:1129–1135, 1986.

40. Sklar CA, Kim TH, Williamson JF, Ramsay NKC: Ovarian function after successful bone marrow transplantation in postmenarcheal females. Med Pediatr Oncol 11:361–364, 1983.

41. Sanders JE, Buckner CD, Sullivan KM, et al.: Growth and development after bone marrow transplantation. In Buckner CD, Gale RP and Lucarelli G (eds): Advances and Controversies in Thalassema Therapy: Bone Marrow Transplantation and Other Approaches. New York: Alan R. Liss, 198, pp 375–382.

42. Rowley MJ, Leach DR, Warner GA, Heller CG: Effect of graded doses of ionizing radiation on the human testis. Radiat Res 59:665–678, 1974.

43. Shaprio E, Kinsella TJ, Makuch RW, et al.: Effects of fractionated irradiation on endocrine aspects of testicular function. J Clin Oncol 3:1232–1239, 1985.

44. Shalet SM, Beardwell CG, Jacobs HS, Pearson D: Testicular function following irradiation of the human prepubertal testis. Clin Endocrinol 9:483–490, 1978.

45. Shalet SM, Horner A, Ahmed SR, Morris-Jones PH: Leydig cell damage after testicular irradiation for lymphoblastic leukemia. Med Pediatr Oncol 13:65–68, 1985.

46. Blatt J, Sherins RJ, Niebrugge D, Bleyer WA, Poplack DG: Leydig cell function following treatment for testicular relapse of acute lymphoblastic leukemia. J Clin Oncol 3:1227–1231, 1985.

47. Damewood MD, Grochow LB: Prospects for fertility after chemotherapy or radiation for neoplastic disease. Fertil Steril 45:443–459, 1986.

48. Buskard N, Ballem P, Hill R, Fryer C: Normal fertility after total body irradiation and chemotherapy in conjunction with a bone marrow transplantation for acute leukemia (Abstract). 15th Annual Meeting of the EBMT, Badastein/Austria February 26-March 2, 1989.

49. Russel JA, Hanley DA: Full-term pregnancy after allogeneic transplantation for leukemia in a patient with oligomenorrhea. Bone Marrow Transplantation 4:579–580, 1989.

14

Intragenomic DNA Repair: Molecular and Clinical Considerations

Vilhelm A. Bohr, M.D.

Our genetic material is constantly exposed to endogenous and exogenous damage caused by various agents. These agents include irradiation and carcinogens, as well as some chemotherapeutic drugs. This damage can cause malignant transformation, in part via mutations at specific sites in certain oncogenes. Most DNA damage, however, is removed by DNA repair mechanisms. Were it not for these enzymes, we would not survive this exposure. There is good evidence that DNA repair plays an important role in the prevention of cancer. For example, in certain human disorders with high incidences of cancer, the cells are deficient in their capacity to repair DNA damage. Although DNA repair is as essential to the cell as the related processes of replication and transcription, it is not as well understood.

It has been known for about 20 years that deficient DNA repair capacity in individuals can lead to, or at least be associated with, increased cancer risk. Since then, our knowledge about DNA repair in human pathology has grown. DNA repair also appears to be an important parameter in clinical therapy. For instance, enhanced DNA repair has been observed in a number of drug resistant cell lines. It has been proposed that this change in repair is the underlying factor causing the resistance. Drug resistance is an important clinical

problem, and it could possibly be overcome therapeutically by treatment with specific inhibitors of DNA repair, in addition to the drug of choice for the disorder. These examples illustrate the need for further understanding of DNA repair processes and how we may be able to modulate them by drug therapy or possibly gene therapy.

The field of DNA repair has come into focus and there is growing interest in DNA repair among physicians. An important avenue of research involves the cloning of human repair genes, their insertion into hamster cells, and subsequent study of their effects. This can be viewed as an early attempt at gene therapy for DNA repair. Another interesting development in DNA repair (discussed below) is work on the fine structure of intragenomic heterogeneity of the repair processes. These advances have been made possible by the development of molecular methods to study DNA repair processes in individual genes. We will also discuss the status of the work on gene-specific repair. Obviously, the advances in understanding DNA repair will have important molecular and clinical implications. It is no longer sufficient to determine DNA repair as an average over the entire cellular DNA; the repair efficiency is heterogeneous over the genome. When we correlate DNA repair capacity to clinical parameters or to biological endpoints, it is increasingly evident that we must also examine the repair process at the level of the individual gene.

DNA DAMAGE

A large number of compounds and agents are known to cause direct damage to DNA. The damage can be changes or alterations of the bases, intrastrand or interstrand cross-links, strand breaks, and incorporation of bulky adducts. Ionizing radiation causes strand breaks and base modifications. Ultraviolet (UV, 254 nm) irradiation induces a number of different types of damage (photoproducts) in DNA. The most common of them is the pyrimidine dimer, a covalent linkage between two adjacent pyrimidines.

Many chemotherapeutic agents cause direct damage to DNA and this damage is often responsible for the cytotoxicity of the drug.

Alkylating agents include many clinically useful drugs that bind covalently to DNA; examples are nitrogen mustard, cyclophosphamide, ifosfamide, melphalan, chlorambucil, and busulfan. Bifunctional agents can form cross-links in DNA. Monofunctional and bifunctional nitrosoureas used in clinical practice include streptozotocin, bischlorethylnitrosurea (carmustine, BCNU), cyclohexylnitrosurea (lomustine, CCNU), and methycylohexylnitrosurea (semustine, methyl CCNU). The alkylation at the N^7 position of guanine is the predominant product, but the O^6 position of guanine can also be modified by alkylating agents and represents another important target for these compounds. Many other base modifications are possible and the spectrum varies for each specific agent.

Cis-platinum (II) diamminedichloride (cisplatin) and carboplatinum are heavy metal compounds with antitumor activity. Covalent bonds are formed with DNA and both intrastrand and interstrand cross-links occur. The most frequently recognized base sequences are GG, AG, and GNG (when N is any nucleotide), but interstrand cross-links only account for about 1% of the damage.

Antitumor antibiotics such as bleomycin bind preferentially to GT or GC sequences and produce free radicals that result in single and double-strand breaks in DNA. The anthracyclines, daunomycin and adriamycin, cause single-strand DNA breaks probably through interaction with DNA topoisomerase II. Mitomycin C, another antitumor antibiotic, acts as a DNA intercalating agent after activation by the cell and can cross-link DNA. Actinomycin D inhibits RNA and DNA synthesis and causes single-strand breaks after intercalation into DNA. The epipodophyllotoxins, etoposide (VP16), and teniposide (VM26), can cause single- and double-strand breaks in DNA through their interaction with topoisomerase II.

DNA REPAIR MECHANISMS

Cells exposed to damage deal with it in different ways. In some cases they simply tolerate or live with the damage. This tolerance is an important pathway that is still poorly understood and that often involves damage bypass replication and introduction of errors in daughter DNA. Recombination processes can be categorized both under tolerance and repair pathways.

DNA damage can be directly reversed only under a limited number of circumstances. These circumstances include the direct removal of UV-induced pyrimidine dimers by photolyase, as well as O^6-alkylguanine damage from various alkylation agents, which can be directly repaired by the mammalian O^6-alkyltransferase enzyme. More often, the elaborate nucleotide excision repair mechanisms are involved; this is the most general and widely characterized form of DNA repair. The sequential steps in nucleotide excision repair include: 1) preincision recognition of damage, 2) incision of the damaged DNA strand near the site of the defect, 3) excision of the defective site and localized degradation of the affected strand, 4) repair replication to replace the excised region with a corresponding stretch of normal nucleotides, and 5) ligation to join the repair patch at its 3 end to the contiguous parental DNA.

The enzymes involved in DNA repair can be classified according to their role in the steps outlined above. Recognition of the damage and incision may be carried out by the same enzyme. An example of this is the pyrimidine dimer specific endonuclease, T4 endonuclease V from bacteriophage T4 infected *Escherichia coli* (E. coli). It has a combined glycosylase and AP endonuclease activity resulting in cleavage of the DNA strand at sites of pyrimidine dimers. In *E. coli*, the repair process can also be carried out by the ABC excinuclease enzyme complex, which consists of three high molecular weight gene products. The ABC excinuclease enzymes recognize a large number of bulky adducts in DNA [1]. The enzyme complex nicks the DNA strand at both sides of the adduct, and in most cases removes a stretch of 12 bases containing the adduct. It is possible, but not established, that a similar enzyme complex to ABC excinuclease is present in eukaryotic cells. Whereas many of the enzymes involved in DNA repair have been characterized in bacteria, only a few of those involved in mammalian repair are known.

MEASUREMENTS OF DNA REPAIR

A number of different methods to measure DNA repair have been developed over the years [2]. A simple method involves determination of the loss of radioactively labeled adducts.

The adducts in DNA can also be directly identified by various methods. DNA re-

pair activity after UV light damage has been determined by a number of different techniques measuring one or more of the aforementioned steps of the repair process. The repair can be measured as the ligation of DNA strand breaks, for example, by using alkaline elution or alkaline sucrose gradient analysis of DNA, or by methods that assess the unwinding of DNA caused by the formation of strand breaks. The polymerization step of the repair process may be measured by unscheduled DNA synthesis or repair replication.

DNA REPAIR AT THE LEVEL OF THE GENE

It is well recognized that DNA in the nucleus of mammalian cells exists as chromatin, which is organized and packaged into higher order structures. This highly complex structural organization must affect all nuclear reactions including replication, transcription, recombination, and DNA repair. The mammalian genome contains on the order of 10^5 genes that constitute about one percent of the total DNA, the remainder being noncoding sequences. Techniques have recently been developed to study damage and repair in genes and other specific sequences [3–5]. In general, this approach can be used to determine the frequency of strand breaks in any genomic restriction fragment of interest. A requirement is that a strand break can be generated at the site of the DNA damage. This is accomplished in different ways for different kinds of damage. Some agents cause strand breaks directly (e.g., ionizing radiation and bleomycin) and in other cases the DNA lesions are detected with specific endonucleases that cleave the DNA or (for alkylation) after depurination are followed by alkaline hydrolysis. The frequency of strand breaks in specific restriction fragments is determined through quantitative Southern analysis and probing of denaturing gels. The technique is outlined in Figure 1 and will now be briefly discussed. Cells are uniformly prelabeled with [³H]thymidine to tag the DNA. After damage the cells are incubated for repair in the presence of the heavy thymidine analog bromodeoxyuridine (BrdUrd); this allows us later to separate the (semiconservatively) replicated DNA from the parental. This step is required in most repair experiments since the replicated (lesion free) DNA can mistakenly be assayed as repaired. The DNA is then isolated, restricted, and the parental DNA is separated on CsCl gradients. After DNA quantitation, strand breaks are generated by endonuclease treatment or (for alkylation) depurination followed by alkaline hydrolysis, and the DNA is elec-

trophoresed on alkaline gels. After transfer, the membranes are hybridized with appropriate DNA probes and subjected to autoradiography. Bands are quantitated by densitometry or directly on the membrane using a (Betagen) blot analyzer. The number of lesions per fragment is calculated from the zero class, that is, the fraction of fragments free of damage, using the Poisson distribution. Initially, a specific endonuclease (T4 endonuclease V) was used to detect pyrimidine dimers after UV irradiation. It is now possible to use the bacterial enzyme ABC excinuclease to detect the DNA damage and repair of bulky adducts other than pyrimidine dimers in specific genes. Damage and repair in specific genes can be studied after

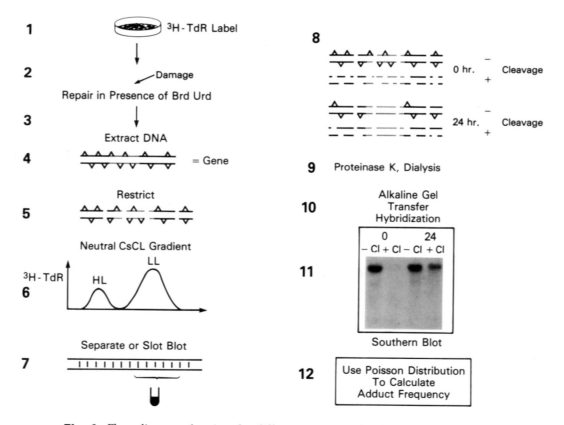

Fig. 1. Flow diagram showing the different steps involved in measurements of gene-specific DNA repair. The protocol is discussed in the text.

TABLE 1. Strand Breaks at Sites of Damage

Type of damage	Cleavage
UV irradiation	
Pyrimidine dimers	T4 endonuclease V
6–4 photoproducts	Photolyase + ABC excinuclease
Cisplatin	ABC excinuclease
Quinoline	ABC excinuclease
NAAAF[a]	ABC excinuclease
Alkylation damage	Depurination + alkaline hydrolysis

[a]NAAAF = N-acetoxy-2-acetylaminofluorene

treatment of cells in culture with various agents that are recognized and incised by the ABC excinuclease. The purified DNA is then reacted with the excinuclease to create strand breaks at sites of DNA damage. In another approach, strand breaks at sites of alkylation are generated by depurination followed by alkaline hydrolysis. These three different approaches are listed in Table 1.

PREFERENTIAL DNA REPAIR IN ACTIVE GENES

Most available results on gene-specific repair have been obtained after UV damage. It was initially shown that repair of UV damage in the essential gene for dihydrofolate reductase (DHFR) in Chinese hamster ovary (CHO) cells is much more efficient than the repair in the overall genome [3]. In normal, repair proficient human cells, the whole genome is repaired during 24 hr after UV damage. However, essential genes are repaired *faster* than noncoding sequences in the genome [6]. This phenomenon has been termed *preferential DNA repair*. Repair has been examined in many different genes, and in cells of a variety of different species. The data suggest that the preferential DNA repair of pyrimidine dimers in active genes after UV damage is not only a general phenomenon in mammalian cells, but is also present in species as diversified as goldfish, yeast, and *E. coli*.

ONCOGENES, REPAIR, AND TRANSCRIPTION

Different genes within the same cell can be repaired with different efficiencies. In a study on the repair of some protooncogenes in mouse cells, it was found that the *c-abl* gene is repaired much more efficiently than the *c-mos* gene [7]. There are many important differences between these two oncogenes. One is that the *c-abl* gene is actively transcribed in the cells, whereas the *c-mos* is not. These experiments suggest a correlation between the level of transcription and the efficiency of repair in a given gene. This relation was further supported by studies on the repair of UV light damage in the metallothionein gene in CHO cells [8] and in human cells [9]. The repair in the metallothionein gene is markedly more efficient when the gene is transcriptionally active than when it it not. These findings suggest that there is some cellular association between the repair machinery and the transcription machinery.

Preferential DNA repair of genes might be ascribed to the more "open" chromatin structure in actively transcribed genomic regions. The recent demonstration that DNA repair shows strand specificity towards the transcribing strand [10], however, suggests that repair is directed toward certain genomic regions rather than just being dependent on chromatin accessibility. Repair enzymes may be linked with the transcription complex. Further studies are needed to examine the relative importance of features such as the local chromatin structure, the primary DNA sequence, and the function of the DNA sequence for the determination of efficiency and organization of DNA repair.

CHEMOTHERAPEUTICS

Only recently has the range of damage that can be studied at the gene level been expanded to include chemotherapeutic drugs. Of relevance to drug resistance is that we can now detect cisplatinum adducts in specific regions in vivo by use of the ABC excinuclease, and we can also separately visualize the interstrand cross-links in specific genes. The drug treated DNA is denatured (30 mM NaOH for 15 min), allowed to reanneal briefly (10 min on ice), and then electrophoresed. So far, we have found that cisplatin cross-links are repaired much faster from all the regions studied than are the adducts [11]. The cisplatin adducts are preferentially repaired in the active DHFR gene in CHO cells, both when compared to inactive genes, to noncoding genomic regions, or to the overall genome. In the case of alkylating agents, we have studied the formation and removal of nitrogen mustard, dimethyl sulfate, and methyl nitrosourea in specific genes in CHO cells. For nitrogen mustard it appears that there is preferential damage formation in a noncoding genomic region compared to the active gene [12]. This documents that drugs can be preferentially localized in certain genomic regions. It is not clear whether this is related to base composition or sequence of the regions studied or to chromatin structural components. Maybe these assays can be used for gene specific therapy. One could look for therapeutics with high affinity for certain genes such as oncogenes, where the expression may be undesirable in a given disease. Since the desirable effect of some cytostatics is to inactivate genes, we could then obtain this effect at lower drug levels and thus lower side effects.

Whereas dimethyl sulfate is repaired with similar efficiency from an active gene and from a noncoding region, nitrogen mustard and methyl nitrosurea adducts are preferentially repaired from the active gene [12]. Thus, related compounds can be repaired in different ways. We do not yet know how this is regulated, but it is possible that the specific chromatin structural alterations caused by these drugs is the important factor in determining the repair characteristics.

HUMAN DISORDERS AND CANCER RISK

A number of human disorders have been associated with increased DNA damage sensitivity or decreased DNA repair efficiency. As listed in Table 2, they can be classified into those conditions where a DNA repair deficiency has been established, those that may have a repair deficiency, and those that are suspect for a deficiency. For none of these conditions is the etiology of the disease known, nor is it known which precise aspect of the DNA repair mechansim is deficient.

We have analyzed fibroblasts from patients with dysplastic nevus syndrome, Bloom syndrome, Cockayne's syndrome, and various complementation groups of the DNA repair deficient disorder xeroderma pigmentosum for the active gene repair. Cells from patients with these disorders are all hypersensitive to UV damage and have elevated levels of sister chromatid exchanges. The overall genome repair is normal in dysplastic nevus syndrome, whereas in Bloom syndrome a ligase and glycosylase deficiency has been

TABLE 2. Diseases Associated With DNA Damage Hypersensitivity

Disorder	Increased risk of cancer
Documented DNA repair defect	
Xeroderma pigmentosum	++++
Cockayne's syndrome	None
Bloom syndrome	++++
Probable DNA repair deficiency	
Fanconi's anemia	++++
Ataxia telangiectasia	+++
Trichothiodystrophy	None
Possible DNA repair defect	
Dyskeratosis congenita	++
Nevoid basal cell carcinoma syndrome	+++
Retinoblastoma	++++
Neurodegenerative disorders	
Gardner's syndrome	++++
Dysplastic nevus syndrome	++++
Breast cancer	
Alzheimer's disease	
Porphyria	
Secondary leukemia	+++++

described. We examined the repair in the active, essential DHFR gene as well as in the inactive β-globin gene (experiments by M.K. Evans). There was preferential DNA repair after UV light damage in dysplastic nevus syndrome and Bloom syndrome similar to the situation in normal human cells, but it was deficient in Cockayne's syndrome and in most of the xeroderma pigmentosum complemetation groups. The lack of preferential DNA repair in Cockayne's syndrome [13] is of considerable interest, since it is the first demonstration of a human cell line not capable of performing this type of DNA repair. It may mean that Cockayne's syndrome harbors a mutation in a gene that plays a major role in gene-specific DNA repair. This disease thus becomes very interesting as a model for future studies on the clinical role of preferential DNA repair.

It will be important to investigate preferential DNA repair in more of the diseases listed in Table 2 under Category III: Possible DNA repair defect. These are disorders associated with DNA damage hypersensitivity of varous kinds; we have discussed the present state of knowledge about the possible deficiencies in DNA repair in a recent review [5].

There is previous evidence that DNA repair may play a role in protection against chemotherapy invoked cancers. In a study of DNA repair capacity in patients with second tumors after treatment for leukemia, it was found that patients with second malignancies had significantly lower DNA repair capacity than the patients undergoing the same treatment, but not developing secondary cancer [14].

INHIBITORS OF DNA REPAIR

Modulation of DNA repair may become a promising method of circumventing drug resistance. In general, significant DNA damage is accompanied by arrest of the cell cycle in G2. Prolongation of the pre-DNA synthesis G2 phase allows more time for DNA repair prior to DNA replication. Methylxanthines such as caffeine prevent cells from arresting in G2 and, therefore, limit the time available for DNA repair before the cell enters into the S phase. Caffeine also has a myriad of other effects that are not completely understood. For example, in *E. coli*, caffeine has been shown to alter the damage site-specific binding of excision repair enzymes. Whether this occurs in eukaryotic cells in unknown.

Individual DNA repair enzymes may also be inhibited. For example, excision repair pathways may be inhibited by modulation of the repair polymerization step. There are four mammalian DNA polymerases (α, β, γ, and δ). DNA polymerase γ is found only in mitrochondria. DNA polymerase α and δ are mainly involved in DNA replication, but can also play a role in DNA repair in some systems. The main DNA repair polymerase is thought to be polymerase β. Two antineoplastic agents that may inhibit DNA repair polymerase are hydroxyurea and cytosine arabinoside (ara-C). Hydroxyurea inhibits ribonucleotide reductase, which is necessary to maintain an intracellular pool of deoxyribonucleotide triphosphates. Hydroxyurea, therefore, depletes the cell of the building block precursors required to polymerize DNA. Cytosine arabinoside is an analog of deoxycytidine which, when incorporated into DNA, causes chain termination. Although hydroxyurea alone is not generally considered an inhibitor of DNA repair, the combination of both hydroxyrea and ara-C inhibits repair of cisplatin induced DNA damage in a human colon cell line. Another compound, aphidicolin, can inhibit DNA repair by polymerase α and δ, and it inhibits repair of cisplatin adducts in a human ovarian cell line.

PERSPECTIVES

The above was a brief review of the methodology and some results on gene-specific DNA repair. Many DNA-related processes may be directly related to the gene-specific repair. For examples, specific polymerases, topoisomerases, or other DNA-related enzymes could be preferentially involved in the gene-specific repair process rather than in the overall genome DNA repair.

Formation and repair of cisplatin and alkylation adducts can now be detected at the level of individual genes. These chemotherapeutics are frequently used for a wide range of neoplasms and a serious problem often encountered in patients undergoing treatment is the emergence of drug resistance. Multidrug resistance has been widely studied and there seem to be a number of molecular mechanisms involved. Lately, however, there is mounting evidence that DNA repair plays an important role; enhanced DNA repair has been observed in a number of drug resistant cell lines and may be a key parameter in this phenotype. These observations have been made in tissue culture cells, and we still do not know what happens in the patient. There are questions about the repair process that need to be answered in the near future and are approachable with the present technology. Standard tumor cell line screening will not normally identify agents that affect gene specific processes since the genes only constitute about 1% of the genome. The methodology for detection of gene specific damage and repair will also be useful in following patients undergoing therapy. It is likely that damage and repair in certain important genes is a relevant prognostic parameter. From the studies on gene specific damage and repair in mammalian cells after UV light damage, we have learned that the repair of essential genes may be better related to cell survival than is the average overall genome repair [13].

ACKNOWLEDGMENTS

I wish to thank the members of my laboratory group for allowing me to review their unpublished data.

REFERENCES

1. Sancar A, Sancar GB: DNA repair enzymes. Ann Rev Biochem 57:29, 1988.
2. Friedberg EC (ed): In DNA Repair. New York: WH Freeman, 1985.
3. Bohr VA, Smith CA, Okumoto DS, Hanawalt PC: DNA repair in an active gene: Removal of pyrimidine dimers from the DHFR gene of CHO cells is much more efficient than the genome overall. Cell 40:359–369, 1985.
4. Bohr VA, Okumoto DS: Analysis of frequency of pyrimidine dimers in specific genomic sequences. In Friedber EC and Hanawalt PC (eds): DNA Repair: A Laboratory Manual of Research Procedures (Volume 3). New York: Marcel Dekker, 1988, pp 347–366.
5. Bohr VA, Evans MK, Fornace A Jr: DNA repair and its pathogenetic implications. Lab Investigation 61:143–161, 1989.
6. Mellon I, Bohr VA, Smith CA, Hanawalt PC: Preferential DNA repair of an active gene in human cells. Proc Natl Acad Sci USA 83:8878–8888, 1986.
7. Madhani HD, Bohr, VA, Hanawalt PC: Differential DNA repair in transcriptionally active and inactive proto-oncogenes: c-abl and c-mos. Cell 45:417, 1986.
8. Okumoto DS, Bohr VA: DNA repair in the metallothionein gene increases with transcriptional activation. Nucleic Acids Res 15:10021–10029, 1987.
9. Leadon SA, Snowden MM: Differential repair of DNA damage in the human metallothionein gene family. Mol Cell Biol 8:5331–5339, 1988.
10. Mellon IM, Spivak G, Hanawalt PC: Selective removal of transcription-blocking DNA damage from the transcribed strand of the mammalian DHFR gene. Cell 51:241–246, 1987.
11. Jones JC, Zhen W, Reed E, Parker R, Sancar A, Bohr VA: Gene-specific formation and repair of cisplatin intrastrand adducts and interstrand crosslinks in CHO cells. J Biol Chem 266:7101–7107, 1991.
12. Wassermann K, Kohn K, Bohr VA: Heterogeneity of nitrogen mustard induction and repair at the level of the gene following treatment of CHO cells. J Biol Chem 265:13906–13913, 1990.
13. Venema J, Mullenders LH, Natarajan AT, van Zeeland AA, Mayne LV: The genetic defect in Cockayne syndrome is associated with a defect in repair of UV-induced DNA damage in transcriptionally active DNA. Proc Natl Acad Sci USA 87:4707–4711, 1990.
14. Bohr VA, Koeber L: DNA repair in lymphocytes from patients with secondary leukemia as measured by strand rejoining. Mutat Res DNA Repair 146:219–225, 1985.
15. Bohr VA, Okumoto DS, Hanawalt PC: Survival of UV-irradiated mammalian cells correlates with efficient DNA repair in an essential gene. Proc Natl Acad Sci USA 83:3830–3833, 1986.

15

Genetic Counseling for the Cancer Survivor: Possible Germ Cell Effects of Cancer Therapy

John J. Mulvihill, M.D., and Julianne Byrne, Ph.D.

Approximately 45,000 individuals are survivors of childhood cancer from the years 1955–1982 [1]. Based on national cancer incidence data [2], we estimate that each year, 65,700 persons under the age of 45 will develop cancer. In addition, there are many individuals in their reproductive years who receive cytostatic treatment for organ transplantation, kidney disease, and other autoimmune disorders, perhaps several thousand a year. Questions are being asked regarding the effects of these treatments on human reproduction. The potential toxic effects of cancer therapy on reproduction include neuroendocrinological and genital tract effects, psychosexual consequences, and the possibility of mutation of the germ cells. Definitive answers are not in hand for any of these areas. Only the dilemma of possible genetic damage is addressed here, including our suggestions for genetic counseling in 1990.

THEORETICAL CONCERNS

Part of the dilemma is that the agents used to treat cancer are specifically designed to interfere with DNA and cellular metabolism, and with cell division. There is good reason to suspect they will cause mutation and genetic disease in human beings.

Standard assays of the mouse at the Oak Ridge National Laboratory [3] show a linear dose–response curve for ionizing radiation as a cause of germ cell genetic damage at several loci. The Oak Ridge Laboratory has generated the experimental results used to set guidelines for radiation protection, specifically for germ cell effects in human populations. The data are based on just a few loci in a laboratory species and they may not reflect directly the sensitivity of the human organism. For example, species may differ in their capacities to repair damage to germ cell DNA following environmental exposures.

Cancer treatments certainly cause genetic damage to somatic cells in human beings. After all, some modern treatment cause cancer themselves and, at the level of the cell, cancer is a genetic disease. Also, cytogenetic abnormalities are commonly seen after intensive cancer therapy. The problem is that though there is considerable information about somatic effects in experimental systems, some data about germ cell effects in experimental animals, and much information about somatic cell mutation in human beings, little is known about the sensitivity of the human gonad to mutagens. Dose-dependent abnormalities have been shown in meiotic chromosomes of the human testes after experimental radiation; to date, how-

Late Effects of Treatment for Childhood Cancer, pages 113–120 © 1992 Wiley-Liss, Inc.

ever, no environmental agent has been causally linked to human germ cell mutation. Yet, in genetic counseling, in the area of mutagenicity of the human gonad, the ultimate measure of concern is human hereditary disease. Does cancer treatment cause hereditary damage in human beings? Does it cause actual disease in the offspring, or mutational events without clinical significance? In theory, the effects of mutation may be neutral or even beneficial, as an essential element of biologic evolution.

The atomic bomb survivors in Japan have been extensively studied for possible genetic damage to their offspring [4,5]. The data are limited, but are compatible with the interpretation that human germ cells may be much more tolerant of ionizing radiation than the standard laboratory mouse. In the most recent definitive summary, Neel states, "We found no clearly statistically significant effects of parental exposures on the offspring characteristics which we studied, but the various indicators of possible genetic damage all are in the direction expected if an effect were indeed produced [6]." A more recent evaluation of the same data suggests that the dose required to double the spontaneous mutation rate in human beings is five times greater than the dose in the mouse [5]. In other words, human germ cells may be five times more resistant to the same dose of radiation than the mouse.

The offspring of the Japanese survivors were studied for eight indicators of possible genetic damage: untoward pregnancy outcome (including congenital malformations), survival of liveborn infants, balanced structural rearrangements of chromosomes, sex chromosome aneuploidy, sex ratio among children of exposed mothers, altered protein charge or function, malignant neoplasms, and growth and development. None of these indicators showed any differences that could be attributed to the parents' exposure. More powerful analysis by two-dimensional protein electrophoresis has been explored, but may not merit full investigation. In addition, there are a number of candidate assays of DNA to see whether or not the DNA base change has occurred in an offspring, but none of these is developed to the point of being useful for population screening purposes [3].

GENETIC EFFECTS IN CANCER SURVIVORS

Literature Review

The actual outcomes of pregnancies in survivors of cancer are published as case reports, small series, and some 14 retrospective collections (Table 1) [7]. All the patients had cancer as a child or young adult, most had finished cancer treatment, and then began a pregnancy. Over 844 cancer patients or survivors, nearly four-fifths of them women, initiated a total of 1,761 recognized pregnancies. Of 1,389 liveborn outcomes, only 53 (about 4%) had a major birth defect, a figure that resembles the population rate for such malformations. The range of defects in the 14 studies included common ones such as congenital hip dysplasia, that may, in fact, represent a deformity or the nongenetic extrinsic molding of fetal features. Only three of the disorders were purely genetic diseases, that is, Mendelian traits or cytogenetic defects, as were also, perhaps, the two instances of multiple congenital anomalies. Pendred's syndrome (goiter and deafness) is an autosomal recessive disease, and both parents must have contributed a mutant gene. Hence, it is not certain that therapy caused the mutation. The other two disorders, the possible 18 syndrome and Marfan's syndrome, may represent new mutants but one cannot be confident. Of course, all these studies were hardly comparable and had such relatively small numbers (given the rarity of genetic disease in the general population) that, even in the aggregate, they have low statistical power. With only two instances of possible mutants seen in some 1,400 offspring, experience is obviously limited.

National Cancer Institute Study

To increase the experience (and to address other issues of late consequences of cancer therapy), a team was assembled at the National Cancer Institute (NCI) in 1978 to study the delayed morbidity and mortality in long-term survivors of childhood and adolescent cancer. The collaboration of five cancer registries was enlisted: the Connecticut Tumor Registry, the California Tumor Registry in the San Francisco Bay area, and hopital registries in Iowa, Kansas, and the M.D. Anderson Hospital [21]. Each center was asked to identify individuals with histologically confirmed tumors or clinically diagnosed brain tumors, diagnosis between the years 1945–1975, age 19 years or less at diagnosis, survival for at least five years, and achievement of at least age 21 years by an arbitrary close-of-study date. These criteria provided us with a cohort of long-term survivors of childhood and adolescent cancers who reached an age at which they could be expected to have married and have children.

These criteria emphasizing survival to adulthood produced a very different relative frequency of tumor types than is seen in incidence series available through the U.S. Surveillance, Epidemiology, and End Results (SEER) Program. There, leukemia, brain tumors, and Hodgkin's disease predominate in childhood and adolescence. Our predominant tumor types were Hodgkin's disease, followed by brain tumors, thyroid carcinoma, and soft tissue sarcomas, because those were the tumors compatible with long life at the time our

cases were diagnosed. Most were treated by surgery alone and one-third had radiotherapy alone; only one quarter of our cases had chemotherapy.

A questionnaire was administered in person and sometimes by phone, and details were elicited about education and jobs, hospitalizations, infertility and pregnancies, pregnancy outcomes, and health of offspring. There was also a minimal family history and a request for a signed permission for medical records to verify reported tumors, birth defects, infertility, and deaths. Finally, we sought the subjects' permission to contact their siblings, who were asked to serve as controls. Up to two controls per case were identified to account for case-survivors with no siblings.

A preliminary analysis [22] showed that male survivors married slightly less frequently than did male controls, a 10% depression in expected marriage rates. The deficit in rates of first marriage was greatest, 30% among males with brain tumors. We analyzed time from marriage to first pregnancy using Cox proportional hazards modeling [23] and found that fertility was slightly depressed in males, leveling off at about 15% of the rate in male controls. Fertility was only slightly depressed among females. When fertility was examined as a function of the type of treatment received in the first year of diagnosis, individuals (both males and females) treated with alkylating agent chemotherapy and radiation below the diaphragm were most severely affected.

Although fertility rates differed by tumor type and therapy, each case-survivor had an average of about one child who had reached a mean age of approximately 11 years at the time of our interview. Seven cancers were reported in the offspring (five histologically confirmed), compared with 11 in the offspring of sibling-controls (eight histologically con-

TABLE 1. Large Series of Pregnancies in and by Survivors of Cancer[a]

Years[b]	Reference	Exposed parents		Total	Fetal loss[c]	Elective abortions[b]	Total	Liveborn with defects	Types of defects
		Total	Females (%)						
?–1973	[8]	46	63	107	15	3	90	2	Hirschsprung's disease, asymptomatic heart murmur[e]
1956–1973	[9]	58[d]	100	96	18	?	75	3	Pendred's syndrome, tetralogy of Fallot, hemangiomata, eczema and strabismus (one stillborn with aplasia of the anterior abdominal wall)
1944–1975	[10]	48	60	93	12	3	77	6	Amblyopia, autism, scleroderma, rectal stenosis, absent fallopian tube and small uterus, slow learner, foot defect
?–1978	[11]	146	58	286	45	19	236	8	Possibly trisomy 18 syndrome, Marfan's syndrome, deafness, pyloric stenosis, Hirschsprung's disease (same as above), cardiac, brain and multiple malformations
?–1980	[12]	30	77	40	12	10	27	1	Congenital hip dysplasia
1968–1979	[13]	20	100	28	5	5	24	0	
?–1982	[14]	14	57	23	?	?	21	2	Multiple congenital anomalies with mental and growth retardation, panhypopituitarism and cerebral atrophy, gastroschisis

Period	Ref									
?–1973	[15]		24	83	48	3	0	44	1	Pyloric stenosis
1972–1976	[16]		22	100	30	9	4	21	1	Congenital hip dysplasia
1958–1980	[17]		216	100	374	99	36	267	8	Spina bifida, tetralogy of Fallot, talipes equinovarus, collapsed lung, umbilical hernia, desquamative fibrosing alveolitis (two sibs), neonatal tachycardia (plus two anencephalic stillbirths and one sudden infant death)
1965–1983	[18]		?	100	222	58	6	159	5	Not specified
1957–1977	[19]		66	100	87	22	12	53	6	Neurosensory deafness[e], scoliosis and slow learner[e], hydrocephalus[e], cleft lip and palate,[e] hydrocephalus, tracheomalacia
1931–1979	[20]		181	65	246	53	32	190	5	Congenital hip dislocation (two), heart murmur, hypospadias, internal tibial torsion
Total		844	79	1,761	373	132	1,336	53	(4%)	

[a]Modified from [7].
[b]Uncertainty.
[c]Fetal wastage is defined as elective abortion, ectopic pregnancy, spontaneous abortion (miscarriage), and stillbirth.
[d]All gestational trophoblastic neoplasia.
[e]Exposed to cancer treatment during gestation.

firmed) [24]. This represents a slight but not statistically significant excess of cancer in the offspring of case-survivors. In the first five years of follow-up, the children of cancer survivors had three times the number of cancers expected based on rates from the Connecticut Tumor Registry; children of sibling-controls had about one half the expected numbers of cancers. After age five, there is no statistically significant difference. The excess seemed attributable to some hereditary cancers (retinoblastoma, Sipple syndrome, and Wilms' tumor) and to some known syndromes of familial cancer, including elements of the Li-Fraumeni syndrome.

In short, there does not appear to be an overall excess risk of cancer in offspring. What excess risk there was in the offspring seemed to be confined to the first five years of life, and could usually be attributable to a known hereditary syndrome. We have very few person-years of observation in the older adolescent age range, the ages when the majority of our case survivors were first diagnosed with cancer.

Cancer could be one indication of germ cell mutation. For further analyses, we defined genetic disease as a cytogenetic syndrome, a single gene defect, or one of 15 simple malformations tracked for incidence by the Centers for Disease Control, such as neutral tube defects, patent ductus arteriosus, and so on [25].

Potentially mutagenic therapy was defined as radiotherapy below the diaphragm or above the knee and/or chemotherapy with an alkylating agent. Finally, we had to distinguish the known familial cases of genetic versus sporadic disease. Sporadic disease indicated no relative with a similar genetic disease; familial disease meant that there was a relative with a similar genetic disease so that the trait in the offspring was recessive. The overall rate of genetic disease was 3.4% and was not different among the offspring of case-

survivors compared to sibling-controls. Some possible differences in the rates of simple defects in our study groups, compared with population rates, probably arose from artifactual differences in defining the defects and differences in the length of time of follow-up. The case-survivors whose offspring had sporadic genetic disease received potentially mutagenic therapies no more often than did those whose offspring were normal.

Our study of genetic disease in offspring of cancer survivors had an 87% power for detecting a twofold excess, and no such excess was found. The power is deceptive because it mostly orginates from the high background rate of simple birth defects such as ventricular septal defect or cleft lip. One cannot be sure that such sporadic defects represent new mutations because they also might be a result of the polygenic or multifactoral traits that arise from parental genes interacting with environmental factors.

Apart from genetic effects, female survivors may face problems in carrying a pregnancy to term. Higher rates of premature delivery and low birth weight have been documented in several studies [19,20,26] but may be confined to women who had abdominal radiation and were incapable of maintaining a full-term, normal weight pregnancy, perhaps because of uterine fibrosis or vascular compromise.

GENETIC COUNSELING IN 1990

According to a consensus definition, genetic counseling is a communication process that deals with the human problems associated with the occurrence, or the risk of occurrence, of a genetic disorder in a family. This process involves an attempt by one or more appropriately trained persons to help the individual or family: 1) comprehend the medical facts, including the diagnosis, the probable course of the disorder, and the available management; 2) appreciate the way heredity contributes to the disorder and the risk of recurrence in specified relatives; 3) understand the options for dealing with the risk of occurrence; 4) choose the course of action that seems appropriate to them in view of their risk and their family goals and act in accordance with that decision; and 5) make the best possible adjustment to the disorder in an affected family member and/or to the risk of recurrence of that disorder [27].

Genetic counseling of cancer patients in practice will vary depending on when in the course of the disease and its treatment the counseling occurs. At the time of diagnosis, one might first inquire about the hereditary origins of the cancer that the patient has. It is important next to mention that pregnancy is contraindicated during therapy, and birth control should be considered. At the same time, information should be given about the prospects of infertility, the option of sperm banking, and the possibility of healthy children if fertility is preserved.

After therapy ends, which is when counseling is likely to occur, former patients should be told that there are major theoretical concerns about mutational damage and that the actual empirical information in human beings to date is limited. A pregnancy probably should be monitored with ultrasound and the usual indications for amniocentesis. After all, prenatal diagnosis is currently used for lesser levels of anxiety than exist among cancer survivors.

It is important to say that the present results provide some room for reassurance. If there is a pregnancy, the existing data do not indicate a risk of congenital or genetic problems above the 4% risk of a baby with a major malformation that any pregnancy has.

Many questions remain regarding the proper care and counseling of survivors of cancer. Since no center and few nations will, in the near future, have much experience with pregnancies in and by cancer patients, it is hoped that collaborative international studies will prove feasible and will gain wide support from clinicians [28].

REFERENCES

1. Mandelson MT, Li FP: Survival of children with cancer. JAMA 255:1572, 1986.
2. Sondik EJ, Young JL, Horm JW, Gloeckler-Ries LA (eds): 1985 Annual Cancer Statistics Review. Bethesda, MD: National Institutes of Health, 1986.
3. U.S. Congress Office of Technology Assessment: Technologies for detecting heritable mutations in human beings. Washington DC: U.S. Government Printing Office, 1986.
4. Schull WJ, Otake M, Neel JV: Genetic effects of atomic bombs: A reappraisal. Science 213:1220–1227, 1981.
5. Neel JV: Reproduction and genetic effects of gonadal exposure to ionizing radiation in human beings. In Mulvihill JJ and Sherins RJ (eds): Reproduction and Human Cancer. New York: Raven Press, 1988.
6. Neel JV: Genetic effects of atomic bombs. Science 213:1205, 1981.
7. Mulvihill JJ, Byrne J: Offspring of long-time survivors of childhood cancer. Clin Oncol 4:333–343, 1985.
8. Li FP, Jaffe N: Progeny of childhood cancer survivors. Lancet 2:707–709, 1974.
9. Ross GT: Congenital anomalies among children born of mothers receiving chemotherapy for gestational trophoblastic tumors. Cancer 37:1043–1047, 1976.
10. Holmes GE, Holmes FF: Pregnancy outcome of patients treated for Hodgkin's disease. A controlled study. Cancer 41:1317–1322, 1978.
11. Li FP, Fine W, Jaffe N, Holmes GE, Holmes FF: Offspring of patients treated for cancer in childhood. J Natl Cancer Inst 62:1193–1197, 1979.
12. Blatt J, Mulvihill JJ, Ziegler JL, Young RC, Poplack DG: Pregnancy outcome following cancer chemotherapy. Am J Med 69:828–832, 1980.
13. Horning SJ, Hoppe RT, Kaplan HS, Rosenberg SA: Female reproductive potential after treatment for Hodgkin's disease. N Engl J Med 304:1377–1382, 1981.
14. Marradi P, Schaison F, Alby N, et al.: Les enfants nes de parents leucemiques. Nouvelle Revue Francaise de Hematologie 24:75–80, 1982.

15. Bundey S, Evans K: Survivors of neuroblastoma and ganglioneuroma and their families. J Med Genet 19:16–21, 1982.

16. Andrieu JM, Ochoa-Molina ME: Menstrual cycle, pregnancies and offspring before and after MOPP therapy for Hodgkin's disease. Cancer 52:435–438, 1983.

17. Rustin GJS, Booth M, Dent J, et al.: Pregnancy after cytotoxic chemotherapy for gestational trophoblastic tumours. Cancer 288:103–106, 1984.

18. Goldstein DP, Berkowitz RS, Bernstein MR: Reproductive performance after molar pregnancy and gestational trophoblastic tumors. Clin Obstet Gynecol 27:221–227, 1984.

19. Mulvihill JJ, McKeen EA, Rosner F, Zarrabi MH: Pregnancy outcome in cancer patients: Experience in a large cooperative group. Cancer 60:1143–1150, 1987.

20. Li FP, Gimbrere K, Gelber RD, Sallan SE, Flamant F, Green DM, Heyn RM, Meadows AT: Outcome of pregnancy in survivors of Wilms' tumor. JAMA 257:216–219, 1987.

21. Teta MJ, Del-Po MC, Kasl SV, Meigs JW, Myers MH, Mulvihill JJ: Psychosocial consequences of childhood and adolescent cancer survival. J Chron Dis 39:751–759, 1986.

22. Byrne J, Mulvihill JJ, Myers MH, Kalish R, Connelly RR, Austin DF, Holmes FF, Holmes GF, Latourette HB, Meigs JW, Teta MJ, Strong LC: Marriage, fertility and premature meno-
pause in survivors of childhood and adolescent cancer (Abstract). Proc ASCO 6:228, 1987.

23. Byrne J, Mulvihill JJ, Myers MH, Connelly RR, Naughton MD, Krauss MR, Steinhorn SC, Hassinger DD, Austin DF, Bragg K, Holmes FF, Latourette HB, Weyer PJ, Meigs JW, Teta MJ, Cook JW, Strong LC: Effects of treatment on fertility after childhood and adolescent cancer. N Engl J Med 317:1315–1321, 1987.

24. Mulvihill JJ, Myers MH, Connelly RR, Austin DF, Strong LC, Meigs JW, Teta MJ, Latourette HB, Holmes GF, Holmes FF: Cancer in offspring of long-time survivors of childhood and adolescent cancer (Abstract). Proc ASCO 5:216, 1986.

25. Mulvihill JJ, Byrne J, Steinhorn SA, Fokke HE, Myers MH, Connelly RR, Austin DF, Strong LC, Meigs JW, Latourette HB, Holmes GF, Holmes FF: Genetic disease in offspring of survivors of cancer in the young. Am J Hum Genet 39:A72, 1986.

26. Byrne J, Mulvihill JJ, Connelly RR, Myers MH, Austin DF, Holmes GF, Holmes FF, Latourette HB, Meigs JW, Strong LC: Reproductive problems and birth defects in survivors of Wilms' tumor and their relatives. Med Pediatr Oncol 16:233–240, 1988.

27. Fraser FC: Genetic counseling. Am J Hum Genet 26:636–659, 1974.

28. Lyon MF: Measuring mutation in man. Nature 318:315, 1985.

16

Mutation, Segregation, and Childhood Cancer

Stephen G. Grant, Ph.D.

It is becoming clear that most, if not all, cancer has a genetic basis. Moreover, our current understanding of tumorigenesis indicates that somatic events, either classical mutations or segregationlike mechanisms that result in reduction of mutant cancer-predisposing genes to homozygosity, are necessary for the development of cancer. Two types of cellular cancer genes have been identified: the proto-oncogenes and the tumor suppressor genes. The first, and in some cases the only, step necessary for tumor progression resulting from either of these classes of oncogene is mutation. The specific types of mutation necessary are very different between the two classes of oncogene, however. To be involved in tumorigenesis, positive-acting proto-oncogenes must first be activated by a somatic event that leads to unregulated hyperactivity of the gene product. In contrast, the first step towards tumorigenesis involving tumor suppressor genes requires a somatic or germ-line mutation to inactivity, followed by a somatic reduction to homozygosity of the mutant allele.

GENETIC BASIS OF CANCER

The risk of malignant neoplasia is elevated in survivors of primary tumors, especially childhood cancers [1,2]. It has long been postulated that some, if not all, tumors have a genetic basis. Childhood cancers are particularly good candidates for this type of neoplasia since their early onset suggests a genetic predisposition. In the last decade, two types of cancer have been identified that are associated with genetic damage and/or predisposition [3].

One type of cancer is caused by mutation of a specific set of normal cellular genes involved in control of cell growth and differentiation resulting in overexpression or unregulated expression and hyperactivity of the gene product. Usually, only one allele must be affected in this way to promote tumorigenesis; these are therefore dominant cancer-causing mutations.

The second type of cancer involves mutations that result in loss of expression of a second subset of normal cellular genes. In this case, loss of expression implies that both alleles at the gene locus are affected: these cancer-causing mutations are therefore recessive and require a second event to segregate the remaining normal allele before active promotion of cancer occurs.

Even when genetic predisposition is not involved, the treatment of potentially life-threatening primary tumors often mandates the use of treatments that of themselves carry increased risk of secondary neoplasia [1]. These are generally treatments that affect the tumor by causing lethal levels of mutation, discriminating the tumor tissue only by growth kinetics. Agents that are known to have negligible mutagenic capacity may also promote cancer by affecting not the initial

Late Effects of Treatment for Childhood Cancer, pages 121–132 © 1992 Wiley-Liss, Inc.

mutagenic event, but the secondary segregational event that can occur by a variety of mechanisms.

Using the techniques of molecular biology, the spectrum of genetic events associated with carcinogenesis is gradually being determined [4,5]. These mechanisms of oncogenesis invariably involve some type of mutagenic event, either somatic or germinal, and may in addition require one or more subsequent events that can involve mutation, mitotic missegregation, or epigenetic mechanisms.

POSITIVE-ACTING PROTO-ONCOGENES

A causal association between mutagenesis and carcinogenesis has long been assumed; however, only in the last decade has significant progress been made in identifying the underlying genetic basis of some types of oncogenic transformation. Beginning with viral oncogenes, a large number of direct-acting transforming genes have been identified and characterized as mutated homologs of normal cellular genes involved in cell growth and differentiation. These "proto-oncogenes" develop transforming potential only upon overexpression or release from their normal regulatory mechanisms [6]. The over 60 human proto-oncogenes identified thus far [7] include genes for hormones and hormone receptors, intracellular signal transducing proteins, and DNA binding nuclear proteins [8,9].

As these positive-acting oncogenes have been shown to be mutated versions of cellular proto-oncogenes, it is reasonable to assume that both the susceptibility of an individual to cancer and the ability of a treatment or compound to induce cancer might be linked to their mutagenic susceptibility or potential. The types of mutation that result in activation of proto-oncogenes are very specific, however, and difficult to model. The spectrum of mutations that

TABLE 1. Mechanisms of Activation of Cellular Proto-Oncogenes

Mutation
Structural mutation[a] to hyperactivity
Regulatory mutation[a] to overexpression
Regulatory mutation[b] to unregulated expression
Gene amplification
Translocation/inversion/insertion
Proto-oncogene coding regions into heterologous regulatory region

[a]Point mutation.
[b]Point mutation, small deletion or insertion.

might contribute to activation of a cellular proto-oncogene is given in Table 1.

Activated oncogenes have been identified that involve point mutations in proto-oncogenes, which effectively increase the activity of their protein product [10]. Experimental mutation assays, however, have demonstrated that the majority of mutations have the opposite effect upon activity, either significantly reducing activity of the gene or protein or extinguishing it entirely. These data tend to support the hypothesis that random changes are more likely to disrupt the integrity of a gene or protein than improve it. Some proto-oncogene gene products are constructed such that they become active because of a conformational change caused by binding of a signal transducing element. Structural mutations altering the native conformation of the protein or dissociating the active center from a regulatory moiety might also have the effect of conferring unregulated activity and/or hyperactivity.

Point mutations may also activate proto-oncogenes by affecting their transcriptional regulatory sequences. In a simplified model, there are two types of regulatory sequences that might be affected: positive regulators, which are either necessary for expression or act to enhance it, and negative regulators, which act to suppress expression and prevent oncogenic concentrations of the products of cellular proto-oncogenes. By the same reasoning used above for coding sequences, random mutations in positive regulatory sequences compromise the integrity of the sequence, tending to inactivate a gene rather than increase transcription. Random mutations in negative regulatory sequences, however, might be expected to inactivate these functions, allowing the oncogene to be transcribed in an essentially unregulated manner. Thus, point mutations that might activate proto-oncogenes consist of those rare mutations in the coding regions that actually create a more active protein product; those rare mutations in the regulatory sequences that increase the expression of the gene; and those more random mutations in very specific negative regulatory elements that allow aberrant expression of the gene. More extensive genetic alterations such as deletions and insertions would also be expected to be most often deleterious to the gene, and only rarely result in activation or overexpression.

An alternative to proto-oncogene activation by mutation of the regulatory region of the proto-oncogene itself is translocation of the coding regions of the proto-oncogene such that they are under the control of another regulatory region—one that does not have the specific controlling sequences that allow the proto-oncogene to be expressed at the levels appropriate for normal function but does not induce tumor formation. These specific translocations of the coding region of one gene onto the regulatory region of another must necessarily represent a very small proportion of all translocations that do occur, since genes themselves represent a very small proportion of the genome, and in most cases the integrity of either the coding sequences or the regulatory sequences of the translocated genes would be compromised, leading to loss of expres-

sion of both genes. Although rare, this type of proto-oncogene activation has been shown to occur. In one famous example, the coding sequences of the normal cellular c-*myc* proto-oncogene must be specifically translocated into the regulatory region of the immunoglobulin genes to cause Burkitt's lymphoma [11].

The third documented mechanism of activation of cellular proto-oncogenes is gene amplification [12]. In this event, a region of DNA of some arbitrary size is duplicated and reduplicated until many, perhaps hundreds, copies are present. Although these duplication events take place on the molecular level, the magnitude of amplification may be such that the results are discernable cytogenetically. Obviously, should a proto-oncogene be present on the piece of reduplicated material and all or a large number of the copies remain intact and functional, there is potential for overexpression of the gene product. This amplification phenomenon has been observed and studied in cultured cells [13], but the factors that might promote such an event, and indeed the mechanism of DNA amplification itself, is still largely unknown.

RECESSIVE TUMOR SUPPRESSOR GENES

More recently, a second class of genes involved in carcinogenesis has been discovered, variously called "anti-oncogenes," "recessive oncogenes," and "tumor suppressor genes." As these names suggest, it is the loss of activity of these types of oncogenes that is associated with carcinogenesis. This type of cancer was first identified through the unusual kinetics associated with the development of retinoblastoma, a childhood tumor of the eye [14]. In comparison to proto-oncogenes, the study of tumor suppressor genes is in its infancy, and the prototypic recessive oncogene remains the retinoblastoma susceptibility gene on chromosome 13. Due to their mode of action, it has been suggested that the normal function of recessive oncogenes is to act as negative regulators of cellular proto-oncogenes [3]. This hypothesis is consistent with the characteristics of the protein product of the retinoblastoma susceptibility locus, which has been cloned [15–17]. The retinoblastoma protein forms stable complexes with the oncogenic proteins of several mammalian DNA viruses, including adenovirus, papilloma viruses, and SV40 [18–20]. It also has several characteristics of a cell cycle regulatory protein [21], including cyclical phosphorylation and dephosphorylation over the course of the cell cycle [22,23], which may indicate some phase-specific functionality.

Since carcinogenesis is associated with loss of activity of recessive oncogenes, one might expect most cancers to be associated with these loci, since random mutational events are more likely to inactivate rather than activate a gene. As the name implies, however, loss of activity of a single allele of a recessive oncogene does not appear to be sufficient for oncogenesis [24]. Both copies of the recessive oncogene must be lost or inactivated before neoplasia occurs (Fig. 1).

In all cases of tumorigenesis associated with recessive oncogenes, one allele is rendered defective by a classical mechanism of mutation, such as point mutation, insertion, deletion, translocation, or inversion (Table 2). In the hereditary versions of these syndromes, this deleterious mutant allele is inherited or arises spontaneously during meiosis and, depending on the nature of the specific recessive oncogene, all cells in the body are at risk for subsequent events that might allow phenotypic expression of the mutant allele and promote neoplasia. In sporadic or nonhereditary cases, both events must take place in the same cell and in a defined order, first an inactivating mutation, then,

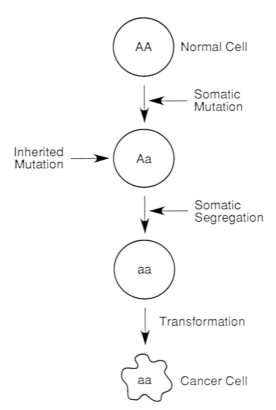

Fig. 1. Two-hit theory of recessive oncogenesis. In the first step, a normal somatic cell with a wild-type genotype at some putative recessive oncogene, A, loses expression of one allele of this locus via somatic mutation. Alternatively, the deleterious allele is inherited as a germinal mutation. This heterozygous cell then undergoes allele loss or reduction to homozygosity at this locus by mechanisms that include mutational, epigenetic, and chromosomal events, summarized as somatic segregation.

in a clonal derivative of that mutant cell, the secondary event allowing expression of the oncogenic phenotype. Obviously, individuals manifesting a recessive cancer of the sporadic type are at much lower risk for multiple, bilateral, or recurrent tumors.

The fact that sporadic recessive tumors occur at all, however, especially in childhood, has two important implications. First, the manifestation of a mutation at a single tumor suppressor locus may be sufficient for tumorigenesis. Second, the frequency of events contributing to this type of cancer are higher than might be implied by mutagenesis studies. As a rough figure the frequency of inactivating mutation at the X-linked HPRT locus both in vivo and in vitro is approximately 10^{-6} [25,26]. Thus, if mutation is the only event contributing to oncogenesis, the frequency of recessive tumors should be $10^{-6} \times 10^{-6} = 10^{-12}$. The mechanism of the second event is less restricted, however, since a second mutation is not strictly necessary, merely an event that allows expression of the first mutation. Appropriate mechanisms, therefore, include not only classical mutagenic events, but also chromosomal missegregation events that allow expression of the recessive phenotype, cancer, associated with the mutant allele [27]. Such missegregation events, resulting in effective loss of one copy of a chromosome or large cytogenetically detectable deletions, were long thought to be inconsequential in vivo, since such cells should be inviable or at a selective disadvantage with respect to their wild-type neighbors, by analogy with the uniform lethality of meiotic monosomies. Oncogenic transformation, however, at least on the cellular level, is an advantageous phenotype, and can overcome the deleterious effects associated with aneuploidy and single chromosome monosomy. Thus, chromosome loss as a secondary event after

TABLE 2. Mechanisms of Mutation of Recessive Tumor Suppressor Genes

Structural mutation[a] to inactivity

Regulatory mutation[a] to nonexpression

Mutation[a] affecting mRNA processing or stability

Gene deletion

Translocation/inversion disrupting integrity of the gene

[a]Point mutation, small deletion or insertion.

mutagenesis has been documented in recessive tumors [28,29].

Although simple somatic chromosome loss has been demonstrated in recessive tumors, another chromosomal loss mechanism involving in situ dosage compensation for the reduction to hemizygosity of genes on the chromosome of interest occurs more frequently. In this event, not only is the chromosome carrying the wild-type oncogenic locus lost, but there is an associated reduplication of the mutant homolog. This type of loss and duplication event was first demonstrated using cytogenetic markers in cell culture systems [30–33] and confirmed in human recessive tumors using Southern hybridization of polymorphic molecular probes [27–29,34–38]. The molecular basis of this event has generally been presumed to be missegregational, either a succession of two nondisjunctions or a concerted loss and duplication in a single aberrant disjunction. The former explanation requires that three independent events occur in the same cell or clonal cell population before tumorigenesis can result—a mutation followed by two nondisjunctions. If the nondisjunction events are indeed independent, then the frequency of such cells should be correspondingly low. On the other hand, a concerted event would imply some connection between the two chromosomal homologs during mitotic segregation (as occurs during meiotic segregation), which is contrary to current evidence. Probably the best explanation is that chromosome loss occurs first, beginning the tumorigenic process, but cells that subsequently duplicate their remaining homolog have a greater probability of surviving and forming a tumor. This is consistent with the presence of variants with apparent deletion of a significant proportion of one chromosome, but not complete chromosome loss, accompanied by reduplication of the homolog in the in vitro model [33].

TABLE 3. Known Segregational Mechanisms of Two Recessive Cancers and an In Vitro Model of Allele Loss

Gene	Chromosome deletion	Chromosome loss	Loss and duplication	Gene inactivation[a]	Mitotic recombination	Total
Retinoblastoma	0	1	6	7	2	16
Osteosarcoma	0	0	8	7	0	15
RB-1 (human chromosome 13)	0	1	14	14	2	31
Wilms' tumor	1	1	10	10	1	23
Hepatoblastoma/rhabdomyosarcoma	0	0	4	2	0	6
WAGR (human chromosome 11)	1	1	14	12	1	29
emtB, chr (Chinese hamster chromosome 2)	21	14	116	46	2	199

[a]Including true gene inactivation as well as point mutation, small deletion, gene conversion, and other mechanisms that do not lead to allele loss at flanking markers.

A second mechanism of reducing a locus to homozygosity without effective loss of genetic material is mitotic recombination. A recombinant event between the centromere and the gene of interest will result in 50% daughter cells that are partial homozygotes (based on random chromosome segregation at mitosis); one-half of these will be homozygous for the mutant allele. Again, this mechanism was first demonstrated in a cell model system [39], then subsequently found to contribute to recessive oncogenesis [27,29,35–38].

Obviously, the disadvantageous consequences of these chromosomal mechanisms can be avoided if the secondary event affects only the recessive oncogene. Thus, the classical mechanisms of point mutation, insertion, and deletion may account for loss of expression of the second allele as well, through a second mutagenic event independent of the first, predisposing mutation. The wild-type gene need not be itself mutated, however, merely rendered unable to complement the oncogenic phenotype of the primary mutation. Thus, there is evidence for contributing epigenetic events such as gene inactivation associated with allele-specific DNA methylation [40,41] and genomic imprinting [42,43], although definitive demonstration of this mechanism has occurred only in cell culture systems [33,44].

Collectively, we have defined this spectrum of secondary oncogenic events as "segregational" mechanisms [45] because they all effectively separate or segregate the recessive mutant allele from its complementing wild-type homolog, allowing expression of the oncogenic phenotype. Since there are many such mechanisms, if any or all occur at frequencies at or above that of mutation, they should act to increase the frequency of secondary events in recessive cancers. In cell culture, the frequency of such segregation events is 10^{-3}, several orders of magnitude higher than simple mutation [30,31,33]. In the best in vivo human somatic model, these segregation events occur at a frequency of 2×10^{-5}, still somewhat higher than mutation frequency [46]. The high frequency of the second event in recessive mutagenesis, coupled with the assumption that only classical mutational events were involved, has led in the past to the hypothesis that the rate of occurrence of subsequent events in tumorigenesis is affected by the first or previous events; that is, oncogenes might have some "mutator" effect. Clearly, this is not the case with the oncogenes characterized thus far, and furthermore, the existence of alternate pathways and mechanisms for tumorigenic progression, such as the segregational events described above, bring into the question the necessity of invoking unusual high-frequency mutational mechanisms.

A comparison of the specturm of events documented for two known recessive cancers, retinoblastoma and Wilm's tumor, with the best studied cell culture model is given in Table 3, and a schematic representation of the known and potential mechanisms of segregation during carcinogenesis via recessive oncogenes is given in Figure 2.

GENETICS AND CHILDHOOD CANCER

Childhood cancers are generally given as examples of cancer with a genetic basis in the traditional sense; that is, they have a hereditary component, implying genetic predisposition to neoplasia. Since we know that most, if not all, neoplasia is caused by mutational and/or segregational events, there are two simple mechanisms for cancer predisposition. The first involves an intrinsicly higher than normal frequency of such events in all somatic cells. This type of predisposition to cancer is clearly demonstrated in individuals suffering genetic deficiencies of DNA repair and/or metabolism [47]. Indeed, the tumorigenic phenotype is so obvious and prominent that such deficiencies are also known as "cancer-prone syndromes." It must be remembered that such a phenotype may also result from environmental influences, which act to increase the frequencies of mutagenic and segregational events such as exposures to radiation or chemicals.

The second mechanism for cancer predisposition in children involves preexisting hereditary lesions, that progress the somatic cells down a tumorigenic pathway. In the simplest case, where tumorigenesis is induced by a single activating mutagenic event at a dominant, positive-acting proto-oncogene locus, it is difficult to envision how such a predisposition could occur, since the entire fetus carries the oncogenic genotype. If such a preexisting genetic mutation was expressed during development, the fetus should never come to term. If, however, the proto-oncogene is expressed in a lineage or cell-type specific manner or is temporally regulated, and such regulation is not compromised by the mutational event itself, neoplasia could result from such a hereditary basis with a very specific etiol-ogy. Thus, cancers that are expressed at a specific time in childhood, such as puberty, or in closely related tissues are good candidates for this type of predisposition.

We are fortunate in that there is a well-studied example of cancer involving a single recessive oncogene, retinoblastoma. As one might expect, genetic predisposition to this neoplasm takes the form of a hereditary mutation at one allele causing loss of activity [48]. Since the phenotype is recessive, there are no direct consequences to carrying such an allele, since it requires a somatic segregational event for the oncogenic phenotype to be expressed. The fact that hereditary retinoblastoma has long been described as a dominant syndrome, indicating the near inevitability of the segregational event, illustrates the high frequency with which such secondary events occur.

These simple models are probably rarely the case in vivo, however. The nature of proto-oncogenes, cell surface receptors and their ligands, and signal transducing proteins and their nuclear effector proteins, indicates that cooperation between these gene products is prob-

Fig. 2. Potential mechanisms of allele loss and loss and duplication at some putative recessive oncogene, A. In the first step towards tumorigenesis, a primary somatic or germinal mutation of the types given in Table 2 inactivates one allele, resulting in a heterozygous cell of genotype A/a, where a represents the recessive inactive mutant allele. In the upper figure four mechanisms of loss of the remaining wild-type A allele are described. These include: a) mutation at the A allele resulting in loss of activity (see Table 2); b) inactivation of the A allele by an epigenetic mechanism such as DNA methylation; c) deletion of an entire region of the chromosome including the A allele; or d) loss of the entire chromosome carrying the A allele. The latter event is shown as occurring via nondisjunction during mitosis, with the simultaneous generation of a daughter cell trisomic for the chromosome of genotype A/A/a. In the lower figure three potential mechanisms leading to homozygosity for the a allele are described, including: a) chromosome loss and duplication, which may occur via two successive nondisjunctional events, or by a single aberrant disjunction in which paired chromatids segregate into daughter cells leading to the generation of both types of homozygous daughter cells, as shown; b) a mitotic recombination event between the centromere and the A locus leading to the indicated daughter cells 50% of the time, depending on chromosomal segregation at mitosis; and c) a putative gene conversion event, in which the DNA from one chromatid is actually replicated by base pairing with the homologous chromosome, with the result that one allele, in this case the A allele, is not replicated at all.

Allele Loss Mechanisms

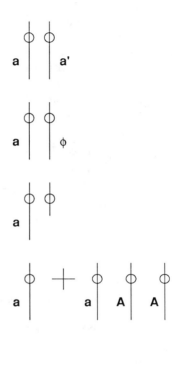

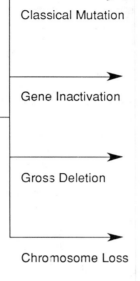

Classical Mutation

Gene Inactivation

Gross Deletion

Chromosome Loss

Allele Loss and Duplication Mechanisms

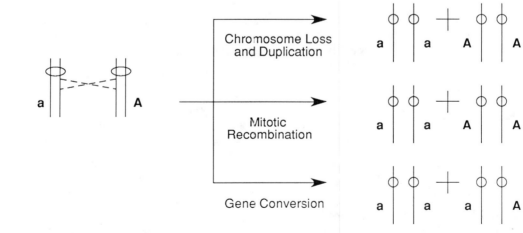

Chromosome Loss
and Duplication

Mitotic
Recombination

Gene Conversion

ably necessary not only for normal cell growth and differentiation but also for most pathways of tumorigenesis. For example, the gene products of the c-*jun* and c-*fos* proto-oncogenes act together to form the transcriptional enhancer/repressor factor AP1 [49], whereas the function of the c-*fms* and c-*kit* proto-oncogenes appear to be redundant, but these genes may be expressed in different, but overlapping spectra of cell types [50]. Thus, multiple mutations activating different proto-oncogenes may be necessary for tumorigenesis. Similarly, the retinoblastoma gene has been implicated in several other neoplasms, notably osteosarcoma and soft tissue sarcoma [51,52]; however, in these tissues other events apparently must contribute before a tumorigenic phenotype is expressed [53]. Perhaps the best model for the true genetic basis of most cancers is the pathway recently proposed for colorectal cancer [54]. The progression of this cancer involves not only activation of the c-*ras* proto-oncogene but also segregation of at least three tumor suppressor genes. If all of these events must occur independently, even if some occur at higher frequency than others, then the progression of such a complicated pathway can be roughly equated with time, which brings us back to childhood cancers as examples of the simplest mechanisms of oncogenesis.

CONCLUSIONS

Elucidating the molecular mechanisms involved in the genesis of neoplasia should have some practical benefit. Thus, in the long term, identification of the specific genes and tumor progression pathways involved in oncogenesis should help treat and ultimately prevent these diseases from occurring. In the short term, however, we can use the general principles we have discovered to be associated with cancer progression, specifically the absolute requirement for one or more somatic mutational or segregational events, to begin to predict and prevent tumorigenesis. Mutagenicity assays have been used in the past to attempt to predict the carcinogenic capacity of exposures to chemicals or radiation, but these assays in general lack the capability to detect segregational events. An assay that incorporates the ability to simultaneously measure both mutagenic and segregational events could be used to detect individuals at risk for childhood cancer because of abnormally high frequencies of these events, and evaluate the capacity of chemicals or treatments, such as those involved in cancer therapy, to induce the events that predispose to neoplasia.

ACKNOWLEDGMENTS

The author would like to thank Ronald H. Jensen, Ph.D., William L. Bigbee, Ph.D., Richard G. Langlois, Ph.D., Barbara R. DuPont, Ph.D., and Jean J. Latimer, Ph.D., for their input and for critical reading of the manuscript. This work was performed under the auspices of the U.S. Department of Energy at the Lawrence Livermore National Laboratory under contract number W-7405-ENG-48.

REFERENCES

1. Boivin J-F: Second cancers and other late side effects of cancer treatment. Cancer 65(Suppl):770–775, 1990.
2. Sanders BM, Jay M, Draper GJ, Roberts EM: Non-ocular cancer in relatives of retinoblastoma patients. Br J Cancer 60:358–365, 1989.
3. Weinberg RA: Oncogenes, antioncogenes, and the molecular bases of multistep carcinogenesis. Cancer Res 49:3713–3721, 1989.
4. Seemayer TA, Cavenee WK: Molecular mechanisms of oncogenesis. Lab Invest 60:585–599, 1989.
5. Hansen MF, Cavenee WK: Retinoblastoma and the progression of tumor genetics. Trends Genet 4:125–128, 1988.
6. Suarez HG: Activated oncogenes in human tumors. Anticancer Res 9:1331–1343, 1989.
7. Trent JM, Kaneko Y, Mitelman F: Report of the

committee on structural changes in neoplasia. Cytogenet Cell Genet 51:533–562, 1989.

8. Herrlich P, Ponta H: 'Nuclear' oncogenes convert extracellular stimuli into changes in the genetic program. Trends Genet 5:112–115, 1989.

9. Knochel W, Tiedemann H: Embryonic inducers, growth factors, transcription factors and oncogenes. Cell Diff Dev 26:163–171, 1989.

10. Bishop JM: Viral oncogenes. Cell 42:23–38, 1985.

11. Croce CM, Klein G: Chromosome translocations and human cancer. Sci Am 252:54–60, 1985.

12. Wolman SR, Henderson AS: Chromosomal aberrations as markers of oncogene amplification. Hum Pathol 20:308–315, 1989.

13. Siminovitch L: Mechanisms of genetic variation in Chinese hamster ovary cells. In Gottesman MM (ed): Molecular Cell Genetics. New York: J Wiley, 1985, pp 869–879.

14. Knudson AG: Retinoblastoma: A prototypic hereditary neoplasm. Semin Oncol 5:57–60, 1978.

15. Friend SH, Bernards R, Rogelj S, Weinberg RA, Rapaport JM, Albert DM, Dryja TP: A human DNA segment with properties of the gene that predisposes to retinoblastoma and osteosarcoma. Nature 323:643–646, 1986.

16. Lee WH, Bookstein R, Hong F, Young LH, Shew JY, Lee EY-HP: Human retinoblastoma susceptibility gene: Cloning, identification and sequence. Science 235:1394–1399, 1987.

17. Fung Y-KT, Murphree AL, T'Ang A, Qian J, Hinrichs SH, Benedict WF: Structural evidence for the authenticity of the human retinoblastoma gene. Science 236:1657–1661, 1987.

18. Whyte P, Buchkovich KJ, Horowitz JM, Friend SH, Raybuck M, Weinberg RA, Harlow E: Association between an oncogene and an antioncogene: The adenovirus E1A proteins bind to the retinoblastoma gene product. Nature 334:124–129, 1988.

19. DeCaprio JA, Ludlow JW, Figge J, Shaw J-Y, Huang C-H, Lee W-H, Marsilo E, Paucha E, Livingston DM: SV40 large tumor antigen forms a specific complex with the product of the retinoblastoma susceptibility gene. Cell 54:275–283, 1988.

20. Dyson N, Howley PM, Munger K, Harlow E: The human papilloma virus-16 E7 oncoprotein is able to bind to the retinoblastoma gene product. Science 243:934–936, 1989.

21. DeCaprio JA, Ludlow JW, Lynch D, Furukawa Y, Griffin J, Piwnica-Worms H, Huang C-M, Livingston DM: The product of the retinoblastoma susceptibility gene has properties of a cell cycle regulatory element. Cell 58:1085–1095, 1989.

22. Buchkovich K, Duffy LA, Harlow E: The retinoblastoma protein is phosphorylated during specific phases of the cell cycle. Cell 58:1097–1105, 1989.

23. Chen P-L, Scully P, Shew J-Y, Wang JYJ, Lee W-H: Phosphorylation of the retinoblastoma gene product is modulated during the cell cycle and cellular differentiation. Cell 58:1193–1198, 1989.

24. Knudson AG: Hereditary cancers: Clues to mechanisms of carcinogenesis. Br J Cancer 59:661–666, 1989.

25. Fuscoe JC, Fenwick RG, Ledbetter DH, Caskey CT: Deletion and amplification of the HGPRT locus in Chinese hamster cells. Mol Cell Biol 3:1086–1096, 1983.

26. Albertini RJ, Sullivan LS, Berman JK, Greene CJ, Stewart JA, Silveira JM, O'Neill JP: Mutagenicity monitoring in humans by autoradiographic assay for mutant T-lymphocytes. Mutat Res 204:481–492, 1988.

27. Cavenee WK, Dryja TP, Phillips RA, Benedict WF, Godbout R, Gallie BL, Murphree AL, Strong LC, White RL: Expression of recessive alleles by chromosomal mechanisms in retinoblastoma. Nature 305:779–784, 1983.

28. Benedict WF, Murphree AL, Banerjee A, Spina CA, Sparkes MC, Sparkes RS: Patient with 13 chromosome deletion: evidence that the retinoblastoma gene is a recessive cancer gene. Science 219:973–975, 1983.

29. Reeve AE, Housiaux PJ, Gardner RJM, Chewings WE, Grindley RM, Millow LJ: Loss of a Harvey *ras* allele in sporadic Wilm's tumour. Nature 309:174–176, 1984.

30. Worton RG, Duff C, Campbell CE: Marker segregation without chromosome loss at the *emt* locus in Chinese hamster cell hybrids. Somatic Cell Genet 6:199–213, 1980.

31. Campbell CE, Worton RG: Segregation of recessive phenotypes in somatic cell hybrids: Role of mitotic recombination, gene inactivation, and chromosome nondisjunction. Mol Cell Biol 1:336–346, 1981.

32. Eves EM, Farber RA: Expression of recessive *Aprt⁻* mutations in mouse CAK cells resulting from chromosome loss and duplication. Somatic Cell Genet 9:771–778, 1983.

33. Grant SG, Campbell CE, Duff C, Toth SL, Worton RG: Gene inactivation as a mechanism for the expression of recessive phenotypes. Am J Hum Genet 45:619–634, 1989.

34. Godbout R, Dryja TP, Squire J, Gallie BL, Phillips RA: Somatic inactivation of genes on chromosome 13 is a common event in retinoblastoma. Nature 304:451–453, 1983.

35. Dryja TP, Cavenee W, White R, Rapaport JM,

Petersen R, Albert DM, Bruns GAP: Homozygosity of chromosome 13 in retinoblastoma. N Engl J Med 310:550–553, 1984.

36. Koufos A, Hansen MF, Lampkin BC, Workman ML, Copeland NG, Jenkins NA, Cavenee WK: Loss of alleles at loci on human chromosome 11 during genesis of Wilm's tumour. Nature 309:170–172.

37. Orkin SH, Goldman DS, Sallan SE: Development of homozygosity for chromosome 11p markers in Wilm's tumour. Nature 309:172–174, 1984.

38. Fearon, ER, Vogelstein B, Feinberg AP: Somatic deletion and duplication of genes on chromosome 11 in Wilm's tumours. Nature 309:176–179, 1984.

39. Wasmuth JJ, Hall LV: Genetic demonstration of mitotic recombination in cultured Chinese hamster cell hybrids. Cell 36:697–707, 1984.

40. Greger V, Passerge E, Hopping W, Messmer E, Horsthemke B: Epigenetic changes may contribute to the formation and spontaneous regression of retinoblastoma. Hum Genet 83: 155–158, 1989.

41. Shiraishi M, Sekiya T: Change in methylation status of DNA of remaining allele in human lung cancers with loss of heterozygosity on chromosome 3p and 13q. Jpn J Cancer Res 80:924–927, 1989.

42. Reik W, Surani MA: Genomic imprinting and embryonal tumours. Nature 338:112–113, 1989.

43. Scrable H, Cavenee W, Ghavimi F, Lovell M, Morgan K, Sapienza C: A model for embryonal rhabdomyosarcoma tumorigenesis that involves genome imprinting. Proc Natl Acad Sci USA 86:7480–7484, 1989.

44. Grant SG, Worton RG: Activation of de novo inactivated genes in somatic cells. Exp Cell Res (in press), 1991.

45. Worton RG, Grant SG: Segregation-like events in Chinese hamster cells. In Gottesman MM (ed): Molecular Cell Genetics. New York: J Wiley, 1985, pp 831–867.

46. Grant SG, Bigbee WL, Langlois RG, Jensen RH: Methods for the detection of somatic mutational and segregational events: Relevance to the monitoring of survivors of childhood cancer. This volume.

47. German J: Patterns of neoplasia associated with the chromosome-breakage syndromes. In German J (ed): Chromosome Mutation and Neoplasia. New York: Alan R. Liss, 1983, pp 97–134.

48. Sparkes RS, Murphree AL, Lingua RW, Sparkes MC, Field LL, Funderburk SJ, Benedict WF: Gene for hereditary retinoblastoma assigned to human chromosome 13 by linkage to esterase D. Science 219:971–973, 1983.

49. Perkins KK, Dailey GM, Tjian R: Novel Jun- and Fos-related proteins in Drosophila are functionally homologous to enhancer factor AP-1. EMBO J 7:4265–4273, 1988.

50. Bernstein A, Rottapel R, Forrester L, Reith AD, Dubreuil P: Molecular genetics of mouse development: Analysis of proto-oncogene mutations in the germ-line (Abstr). Genet Soc Can Bull 21:85, 1990.

51. Hansen MF, Koufos A, Gallie BL, Phillips RA, Fodstad O, Brogger A, Gedde-Dahl T, Cavenee WK: Osteosarcoma and retinoblastoma: A shared chromosomal mechanism revealing recessive predisposition. Proc Natl Acad Sci USA 82:6216–6220, 1985.

52. Weichselbaum RR, Beckett M, Diamond A: Some retinoblastomas, osteosarcomas, and soft tissue sarcomas may share a common etiology. Proc Natl Acad Sci USA 85:2106–2109, 1988.

53. Toguchida J, Ishizaki K, Nakamura Y, Sasaki MS, Ikenaga M, Kato M, Sugimoto M, Kotoura Y, Yamamuro T: Assignment of common allele loss in osteosarcoma to the subregion 17p13. Cancer Res 49:6247–6251, 1989.

54. Vogelstein B, Fearon ER, Hamilton SR, Kern SE, Preisinger AC, Leppert M, Nakamura Y, White R, Smits AM, Bos JL: Genetic alterations during colorectal-tumor development. N Engl J Med 319:525–532, 1988.

Methods for the Detection of Somatic Mutational and Segregational Events: Relevance to the Monitoring of Survivors of Childhood Cancer

Stephen G. Grant, Ph.D., William L. Bigbee, Ph.D.,
Richard G. Langlois, Ph.D., and Ronald H. Jensen, Ph.D.

In the last decade, the new techniques of molecular genetics have gone far towards elucidating the relationship between mutagenesis and cancer. It is now generally accepted that most, if not all, cancer has a genetic basis, and that the progressive steps in multistage carcinogenesis represent genetic mutations and/or a relatively new class of events involving not only classical mutation, but also chromosomal recombination and missegregation events and epigenetic mechanisms. This class of somatic mechanisms is collectively known as segregation, although "reduction to homozygosity," "loss of heterozygosity," and simple "allele loss" have also been used. Childhood cancers, due to their early onset, represent a class of tumors that not only may have the simplest etiology, but may also result from hereditary predisposition to neoplasia.

If the genetic basis of the primary tumor in an individual manifesting such a childhood cancer can be ascertained, it should be possible to determine whether genetic predisposition is indeed involved and, therefore, whether a significant risk of recurrence is indicated. If some type of predisposition to cancer is indicated, an appropriate test or monitoring system might be designed to measure the empirical probability of a recurrence of the molecular events involved in the genesis of that specific type of tumor and, therefore, support reasonable predictions as to the probability, timing, and location of a second neoplasm.

Two general types of genetic predisposition can be postulated. In the first case, the individual is at risk because they manifest a higher than normal frequency of the mutational and segregational events that have been found to contribute to oncogenesis. Alternatively, a germinal mutation can advance the progress of a multistage tumorigenic process resulting in earlier and more frequent manifestation of neoplasia. In the second case, however, there is still an absolute requirement for further somatic mutational and/or segregational events to occur before the oncogenic phenotype is manifested. Thus, on general principles, an assay that allowed quantitation and characterization of such events could be an important diagnostic part of clinical therapy. In practical terms, it would be impossible to simply screen a population with such an assay in order to identify those at risk. In the survivors of childhood cancer, however, there is a significant recurrence risk, higher than the normal population risk of primary neoplasia. This higher risk might simply be due to hereditary factors, the initial tumor serving to identify individuals predisposed to neoplasia. On the other hand, the somatic events that contribute to tumorigenesis may be affected or induced by environmental factors, and the radiation and chemotherapeutic procedures mandated by the primary tumor may actually cause new lesions and create a pool of somatic cells predisposed for tumor progression.

A comprehensive test or monitoring system would also take this mechanism of recurrence into account. Such a monitoring system or predictive assay would ideally be directly applicable to the individual under consideration without unduly complicating or compromising treatment or recovery. In this way, uniquely individual data, probabilities, and predictions can be generated in each case, rather than simply extrapolating from population values.

There is no current assay or modeling system that serves to simultaneously monitor all the possible mechanisms of genesis or recurrence of childhood cancers. Our in vivo human somatic allele loss assay, based upon the erythrocyte-specific cell surface protein glycophorin A (GPA) [1,2], offers the greatest advantages of such assays currently available.

SHORT-TERM ASSAYS OF MUTAGENESIS

The presumed association between oncogenesis and mutagenesis has resulted in short-term mutagenesis assays being performed as indicators of carcinogenic predisposition and potential. The correlation between these two functionalities has not been particularly strong, however. Bacterial tests such as the Ames assay and its many variants require that very specific point mutations occur that reverse the ef-

fects of a preexisting deleterious loss-of-activity mutation [3]. Thus, such tests would appear to be good models for the very specific mutations necessary to activate proto-oncogenes, were there not the uncertainties inherent in extrapolating prokaryotic data to humans. Such reversion assays are not as prominent in mammalian assay systems, however, although they are possible at several loci such as HPRT, APRT, and TK, where in vitro selective conditions have been described that can require either intact enzyme activity or loss of activity for cell survival [4]. The results of such reversion assays, in terms of spontaneous reversion frequencies and response to mutagenic agents, are highly variable, indicating that there may be very different reversion kinetics and mechanisms associated with each independent enzyme deficiency mutation [5]. The implications of these studies for proto-oncogene activation is that activation events will be unique for each locus. Such a spectrum of specific single mutagenic events may well prove impossible to model or assay en masse. Reversion assays rarely involve translocation, another known mechanism of proto-oncogene activation, although reversion by amplification of the deficient allele is not unknown [6,7].

Some relationship is implied between the molecular events involved in chromosomal translocation and those involved in the integration of heterologous genetic material, as both involve illegitimate recombination. There are assays for such activities, for example, the so-called "enhancer-trap" experiments that rely on the incorporation of a transfected reporter gene lacking a promotor into the regulatory regions of an unknown gene for functionality [8]. Indeed, several putative proto-oncogenes have been identified via transformation [9,10] or tumorigenicity [11] assays involving transfection of purified genomic DNA. The activated oncogene identified in this type of assay often arises by illegitimate recombination during the course of the experiment [12–14]. In some cases, such proto-oncogenes, while shown to exhibit transforming potential, have yet to be implicated in neoplasia in vivo.

As a model for the translocational and other recombinational activation events that occur in vivo, a modified enhancer trap assay is necessary. First, a neutral but selectable reporter gene lacking a promotor is stably integrated randomly into the genome of a cell. The resultant cell line is then placed under conditions where the expression of the reporter gene is necessary for survival. In such a system, treatments could be tested for their ability to promote translocation of the reporter gene to a site where it is activated, that is, placed under the control of an active promotor. Genetic mutations affecting mitotic pairing or recombination could also be evaluated for their effect. In a preliminary attempt at such a system [15], rearrangement (tandem duplication) of the integrated plasmid DNA proved to be the only mechanism of activation detected. This assay is therefore limited in its ability to model translocational and recombinational events; nevertheless, the results indicate that the activation event was not affected by known mutagenic agents, and that this particular activation event involved both homologous recombination and gene amplification.

The cytogenetic manifestations of gene amplification, homologously staining regions, and double minute chromosomes, have been equally associated with both in vitro mutation to drug resistance, as well as cancer and the transformed phenotype since their initial discovery [16]. Several in vitro systems have been described in which gene amplification has been shown to occur [17], and the efficacy of treatment with some known mutagenic agents at inducing such events have been evaluated

[18]. Current evidence indicates that gene amplification can be promoted by viral genes [19] or direct DNA damage [20], and may be associated with sister chromatid exchange [21]. At the present time, there is no short-term mutagenicity assay that is designed to simultaneously detect all of these potential mechanisms of proto-oncogene activation.

The only well-established human in vivo assay for mutagenic predisposition or induction is based on loss of activity of the X-linked housekeeping enzyme hypoxanthine-guanine phosphoribosyltransferase (HPRT) [22,23]. In this assay, T-lymphocytes are cultured from human blood and subjected to selection specific for loss of HPRT activity. Random mutations are likely to cause inactivation of the HPRT gene by a wide variety of mechanisms, with little of the specificity inherent in the point mutational activation of proto-oncogenes. As a simple indicator of background point mutational frequency, however, the HPRT assay would be expected to show some association with similar events involved in carcinogenesis. Similarly, the T-cell HPRT assay also roughly measures the frequency of chromosomal events, such as translocation, which can inactivate the HPRT gene. The proportion of translocations that might positively activate a proto-oncogene must be relatively small when considered against the number of random translocations, inversions, and, most importantly, deletions that might inactivate the HPRT gene, however, thus compromising the accuracy of the assay in specifically quantitating these events. Finally, gene amplification has not been implicated as a mechanism of HPRT deficiency, although it has been documented in phenotypic revertants [5–7]. In summary, the activation of proto-oncogenes is a very difficult system to model, and no comprehensive assay is available that measures simultaneously all the possible mechanisms through which such mutations arise, nor do assays exist that require the same specific types of mutations or translocations.

Modeling of the events that contribute to recessive oncogenesis would at first appear to be more straightforward. Functional loss of a gene occurs more often, and should be easier to detect, than gene activation. Thus, the HPRT system described above should, and perhaps does, model the spectrum of point mutations that inactivate mammalian genes, and presumably there should not be any great difference between inactivating HPRT and inactivating a recessive oncogene. This comparison does not, however, take into account the second step in the genesis of recessive tumors, the segregation event. This is the critical step, especially in childhood cancers with evidence of a predisposing germinal mutation, since it can occur by a wide variety of mechanisms. Somatic segregation can be a high-frequency event, potentially disrupting large amounts of genetic material flanking the recessive oncogene by the mechanisms of chromosome loss, deletion, or, in more subtle ways, inactivation or loss and duplication. Segregation may also require the pairing of homologous chromosomes at mitosis in order to occur. This is particularly evident for the mechanisms of mitotic recombination and gene conversion, but may also promote chromosome loss and loss and duplication through aberrant disjuctions and missegregations. When these considerations are taken into account, the initial advantage of the HPRT system—that there is only one functional allele in all mammalian cells and therefore a single mutagenic event is detectable—becomes a disadvantage, by effectively disallowing the most important mechanisms of segregation. Deletion of genetic material from an autosomal locus may have serious consequences, but there remains a second allele on the unaffected homologous chromosome, so that gene

function is not lost entirely. Deletion of material flanking and including the X-linked HPRT gene, however, is likely to be more deleterious since the material lost includes the only functional copies of those genes in the cell. In addition, events that require the exchange of material between homologous chromosomes or involve aberrant segregation of chromosome pairs are restricted with respect to loci on the X chromosome since males have no second X, and the second X in females is irreversibly inactivated. Thus, a new somatic "mutational" assay is required that might incorporate these segregational events into its design.

THE IN VIVO HUMAN GPA MUTAGENESIS ASSAY

The glycophorin A locus was chosen as the basis for a human in vivo somatic cell mutation assay for several reasons. First, for practicality, such an assay should be based on a tissue from which large numbers of single cells can be obtained easily, and preferably noninvasively. Second, for accuracy in estimating individual genetic burden, the assay should be based on an autosomal locus sensitive to a spectrum of mutational mechanisms, from point mutations to chromosomal events, all giving rise to an easily detectable variant phenotype. Third, the assay should be applicable to a substantial proportion of the human population. Finally, for economy and experimental accuracy, the assay should directly detect and rapidly enumerate variant cells.

Erythrocytes were chosen to best satisfy the first condition since a small volume of blood obtained by standard venipuncture can conveniently provide about 10^9 erythrocytes for analysis. The GPA gene, which encodes the most abundant and well-characterized integral membrane sialoglycoprotein on human erythrocytes, was selected as the target locus based on an extensive biochemical and genetics literature indicating that this locus had all of the properties necessary to satisfy the remaining criteria outlined above.

Biochemical genetic data, later corroborated by molecular studies, demonstrated that the GPA gene coded for an erythroid lineage-specific cell surface antigen present at high copy number on the membrane of circulating erythrocytes [24]. The GPA gene is present in single copy in the genome [25], and autosomal localization to chromosome 4q28-q31 has been established by genetic linkage analysis [26] and confirmed by in situ hybridization [27]. The protein coding region of the GPA gene is 453 nucleotides in length, and the genomic structure of the GPA locus has been recently elucidated and consists of seven exons and six introns extending over 40 kB [28]. Thus, the GPA gene is typical in size and complexity for an eukaryotic gene. A central feature of the assay derives from the finding that the GPA gene occurs as two common alleles, GPA^M and GPA^N, that are responsible for the MN blood group. These two alleles are approximately equally represented in the human population [29] and are codominantly expressed in MN heterozygotes [30]. The M and N forms of the GPA protein are identical in amino acid sequence except at positions 1 and 5 from the amino terminus [30,31] where the GPA^M allele has serine and glycine as coded for by TCA and GGT, respectively; on the other hand, the GPA^N allele has leucine and glutamic acid in these positions, as coded for by TTA and GAG [26,32–35].

In individuals of heterozygous MN blood type, there should be rare erythrocytes that fail to present one allelic form of GPA on the cell surface. These phenotypic variants might arise as a result of allele loss-type somatic mutations at the GPA locus in bone marrow erythroid cells, assuming that the mutation was nonlethal, and that erythrocytes with the variant

phenotype were not strongly selected against in vivo. The putative allele loss phenotype should be selectively neutral, based on findings that individuals lacking GPA on their erythrocytes because of an inherited condition are hematologically normal, and their red cells have a normal circulatory lifetime [30,35]. The assay was also designed to require that allele loss variant cells maintain normal expression of the remaining GPA allele, thus eliminating phenocopies and contributions of genetic alterations outside the GPA locus, such as alterations in protein processing, or other epigenetic events leading to loss of presentation of both GPA alleles. Since variant cells of allele loss phenotype are scored, the GPA assay is potentially sensitive to a variety of mutational mechanisms from point mutations, that is, single base substitutions or small insertions or deletions to chromosomal events such as missegregation, aneuploidy, gene inactivation or conversion, and homologous or nonhomologous somatic recombination.

Support for the hypothesis that allele loss at an autosomal locus should occur in vivo came from in vitro studies in mammalian cell systems in which it was demonstrated that spontaneous, chemical- and radiation-induced mutations in polymorphic, heterozygotic loci coding for immunologically distinguishable cell surface antigens result in variant cells of gene expression loss phenotype [36–41]. This work has been recently extended to the development of an in vivo human assay demonstrating HLA allele loss in lymphocytes [42–45]. This assay provides direct confirmation of somatic mutation at the HLA locus in humans in vivo. It is limited, however, in that it requires relatively large volumes of blood, as well as lymphocyte culture and cloning.

Practically, the GPA assay is based on the use of two fluorescently labeled mouse monoclonal antibodies specific for GPA^M and GPA^N to identify rare allele loss variant erythrocytes. Singly labeled variant cells are then rapidly enumerated by flow cytometry and flow sorting to yield the frequency of allele loss variants in the blood of the sampled individual [1,2]. In addition to simple allele loss variants, the in vivo GPA assay has demonstrated that a second distinguishable class of variants exist that have lost expression of one GPA allele and express the remaining allele at a two copy level. These variants occur at a similar frequency to that of the simple allele loss variants [1,2]. Since it is unlikely that such loss and duplication phenotypes can arise by simple mutational events, such variants provide evidence that in vivo somatic segregation occurs at the GPA locus, and probably also contributes to the allele loss class of variants. A summary of possible mechanisms for the genesis of both allele loss and loss and duplication variants is provided in Figure 1.

SECONDARY TUMORS IN SURVIVORS OF CHILDHOOD CANCER

Patients who survive their first incidence of neoplasia are generally at high risk for recurrence. This is particularly true of survivors of childhood cancers, especially those with a genetic basis. Some of the recurrence risk can be attributed to a reemergence of the same primary tumor, either through metastasis or relapse due to regrowth of material not destroyed or removed upon primary treatment. Other than relapse of the original tumor, however, de novo appearance of a new cancer in these patients is usually associated with either a) a new primary tumor resulting from a second, independent segregation event reexposing a genetic predisposition, or b) an entirely new cancer induced by the mutagenic or carcinogenic capacity of the treatment used for the original primary tumor.

Survivors of childhood cancer arising through genetic predisposition are at risk for a recurrence of the cancer because of the same genetic locus. In retinoblastoma, for example, should a child inherit a deleterious allele both eyes are at risk and independent single segregation events continue to be a potential risk after treatment [46]. If the primary tumor was actually of the "sporadic" type, there is less of a chance of recurrence [47] because not all cells in the body are predisposed to this particular locus-specific cancer. Depend-

Fig. 1. Potential mechanisms of allele loss and loss and duplication at the GPA locus on human chromosome 4. In the upper figure four mechanisms of loss of the GPA^M allele are described. These include: a) mutation at the GPA^M allele resulting in either loss of activity or loss of antibody binding; b) inactivation of the GPA^M allele by an epigenetic mechanism such as DNA methylation; c) deletion of a region of chromosome 4 including the GPA^M allele; or d) loss of the entire chromosome 4 carrying the GPA^M allele. The latter event is shown as occurring via nondisjunction during mitosis, with the simultaneous generation of a daughter cell trisomic for chromosome 4 of genotype GPA$^{M/M/N}$. In the lower figure three potential mechanisms leading to homozygosity for the GPA^N allele are described, including: a) chromosome loss and duplication, which may occur via two successive nondisjunctional events, or by a single aberrant disjunction in which paired chromatids segregate into daughter cells leading to the generation of both types of homozygous daughter cells, as shown; b) a mitotic recombination event between the centromere and the GPA locus leading to the indicated daughter cells 50% of the time, depending on chromosomal segregation at mitosis; and c) a putative gene conversion event, in which the DNA from one chromatid is actually replicated by base pairing with the homologous chromosome, with the result that one allele, in this case the GPA^M allele, is not replicated at all.

Allele Loss Mechanisms

Allele Loss and Duplication Mechanisms

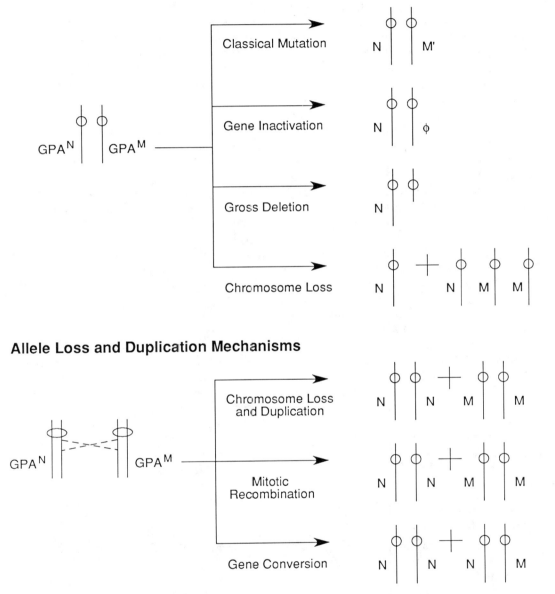

ing on the lag between the first and second "hits," however, there could be a significant population of predisposed somatic cells left in the individual after treatment of the primary lesion. Recurrence does not have to be tissue-specific either. In the case of retinoblastoma, it has long been known that individuals predisposed to retinoblastoma are also likely to develop secondary cancers in other tissues later in life [48–51], notably osteosarcoma and soft-tissue sarcoma [52]. This is because allele loss at the same "retinoblastoma" locus has been shown to be involved in cancer in these tissues as well [53,54]. Thus, the tissues at risk for cancer will probably be different for each recessive oncogene, but will almost certainly involve tissues other than those in which neoplasia first arises.

Retinoblastoma is probably unique in that a single recessive locus appears to be involved in oncogenesis. Most cancers are probably more complicated, involving more than one recessive oncogene [55], and perhaps requiring a combination of events involving both activation of proto-oncogenes and inactivation of recessive oncogenes, as has been partially demonstrated for colorectal cancer [56]. Such tumors will have complicated recurrence kinetics, possibly involving several alternative pathways. Thus, genetic predisposition at a certain locus may have several associated cancers that it can contribute to both directly and indirectly.

RECURRENCE OF A CANCER WITH THE SAME GENETIC BASIS

Recurrence of a cancer resulting from allele loss at the same genetic locus is dependent on the occurrence of a second, independent segregational event resulting in reduction to homozygosity. In predisposed individuals in which the primary tumor is associated with a germinal mutation in one allele, as in the case of "famil-

ial" retinoblastoma, the probability of a second segregational event occurring is dependent on the frequency of somatic segregational events in vivo, which can be measured using the GPA assay [57]. Indeed, the frequency of such events in otherwise normal individuals predisposed to a specific cancer should be indistinguishable from the normal population. The frequency of segregational allele-loss events at the GPA locus in a large population of normal controls from several published [1,2,58] and ongoing studies [59] are given in Figure 2. Since allele loss and loss and duplication events both confer the oncogenic phenotype when they affect a recessive oncogene, the frequency of recurrence depends on the sum of frequencies of these two types of events. Allele loss events occur in our GPA system at a mean frequency of 9.8×10^{-6}, and loss and duplication events at a mean frequency of 9.6×10^{-6} in normal controls from various studies. These normal variant frequencies should be indicative of the frequencies of recurrence of childhood cancers established by epidemiologic studies, since both cancer incidence and GPA variant frequency are measures of directed allele loss. An unusually high GPA variant frequency in such individuals might indicate a correspondingly higher risk of recurrence. Included in Figure 2 are the results of assaying a heterologous group of adult cancer patients after diagnosis but prior to treatment. The results confirm that cancer in these individuals is associated with a normal background frequency of mutational and segregational events, as measured using the GPA assay. Studies are ongoing into the effects of environmental and occupational exposures such as smoking and chemical inhalation on the frequency of variant erythrocytes detected by the GPA assay.

Some patients affected with childhood cancers may be at greater risk for recessive oncogenesis not because they carry a ger-

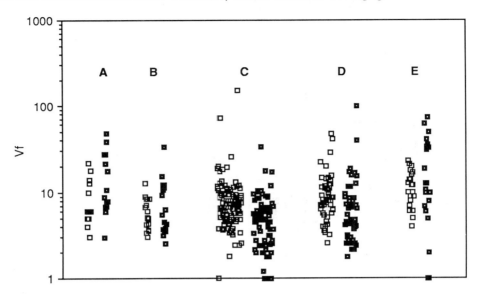

Fig. 2. GPA variant frequencies in normal controls. A summary of background GPA variant cell frequencies per million, Vfs, from several completed and ongoing studies, including: A) an initial set of Lawrence Livermore National Laboratory (LLNL) controls used to develop the GPA assay using a dual beam sorter; B) an overlapping set of lab controls used to develop the assay on the commercially available FACScan flow cytometer; C) controls from an unpublished investigation into the effects of smoking on pregnant women; D) controls from an unpublished investigation into the effects of occupational styrene exposure in Finnish workers; and E) data from patients diagnosed with cancer, sampled prior to therapy.

minal mutation at a recessive oncogene but because their frequency of segregational events is higher than normal individuals. This possibility specifically concerns patients manifesting a sporadic recessive cancer. The most extreme examples of this type of predisposition are the cancer-prone syndromes such as ataxia telangiectasia and Bloom's syndrome, in which a defect in DNA repair and/or metabolism causes a predisposition to cancer [60]. Results of a limited study of individuals suffering from these syndromes examined with the GPA assay are given in Figure 3. Individuals manifesting ataxia telangiectasia show a ten-fold greater frequency of variation by this assay [61]; Bloom's syndrome patients show nearly a 100-fold increase [62,63]. There appears to be a strong correlation between cancer

susceptibility and high GPA variant frequency in these individuals. There was no increase in variant erythrocytes in patients suffering from xeroderma pigmentosum, however [64]. We interpret this result as indicating that susceptibility to genetic damage due to exposure to ultraviolet (UV) light does not increase the risk of mutation or segregation in the erythropoietic precursor cells sequestered in the bone marrow. The magnitude of the response in ataxia telangiectasia and Bloom's syndrome patients suggests that we may be able to discern more subtle effects in individual patients and adjust their probability of recurrence accordingly. Using family studies, we might be able to identify a genetic basis for subtle increases in GPA variant frequencies and, therefore more subtle cancer predispo-

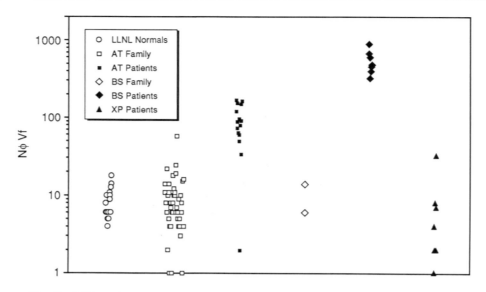

Fig. 3. GPA variant frequencies in individuals suffering from cancer-prone syndromes. Assay results on patients and families of patients with the DNA repair and/or metabolism deficiency syndromes ataxia telangiectasia (AT), Bloom's syndrome (BS), and xeroderma pigmentosa (XP).

sition syndromes. Furthermore, many cancer-prone syndromes are demonstrably heterologous, with complementation groups characterized only by tedious in vitro cell culture methods [60]. The GPA assay may be able to differentiate these complementation groups directly by their differential effects on either or both classes of GPA variant frequencies.

RECURRENCE RESULTING FROM THE MUTATIONAL EFFECT OF CANCER THERAPY

Regardless of genetic predisposition, a second primary tumor can develop as a result of the action of the potentially mutagenic or carcinogenic treatments used on the primary tumor. Under these circumstances, either class of cancer may occur, that is, cancer resulting from the activation of a proto-oncogene or cancer due to allele-loss of a recessive oncogene, since both classes involve mutational events. As mentioned earlier, there is presently no

adequate model for the mechanisms involved in activating a proto-oncogene. Two of these mechanisms occur by events that might also contribute to allele loss, point mutation and translocation. The rationale behind the HPRT assay is that a measure of the overall frequency of mutations inactivating the HPRT gene should bear some relationship to the frequency of mutagenic events capable of activating proto-oncogenes. This same rationale can be applied to the GPA assay; indeed, the GPA assay should provide a more accurate measure of mutagenic events since, unlike variants lacking HPRT activity [65], null variants at the GPA locus are at no obvious disadvantage relative to their neighbors and are not selected against. In addition to mutagenic events, the GPA assay is sensitive to segregational mechanisms contributing to allele loss that may occur at higher frequencies than classical mutation.

We have investigated the effects of whole-body ionizing radiation upon the frequency of variants at the GPA locus in three studies: survivors of the bombing of Hiroshima [66,67]; survivors of the accident at the Chernobyl nuclear reactor [64]; and survivors of an accident with a ^{137}Cs source in Goiania, Brazil [68]. The results of these studies are summarized in Figure 4. A similar dose-dependent increase in the frequency of variant erythrocytes was observed in all three cohorts. In contrast, preliminary results on samples from cancer patients treated by fractionated doses of ionizing radiation indicate little, if any, response to this treatment using the GPA assay [69]. We believe this is a function both of the very high localized dose (12–50 Gy), which predominantly kills rather than mutates erythropoietic bone marrow stem cells, and the small area of irradiation, which exposes only a fraction of the total stem cells present in the marrow. We anticipate that our assay will be more applicable to radiotherapy involving ^{131}I or radioimmunotherapy, where the injected radioisotope is dispersed in the bloodstream prior to localization, resulting in a significant exposure to the entire erythroid bone marrow.

Often, constituents of cancer chemotherapy are themselves mutagenic or carcinogenic, and these potentialities may be detected with the GPA assay [58]. Figure 5 demonstrates two extremes of the responses we have observed in patients following chemotherapy with such agents. In a population of breast cancer patients undergoing CAF adjuvant chemotherapy, a large initial response was observed, but there was little evidence of long-term persistence of elevated therapy-induced variant frequencies. These data suggest that the mutagenic components of this therapy, adriamycin and cyclophosphamide, predominantly induce mutations in the dividing and differentiating cells of the erythropoietic lineage, but produce little

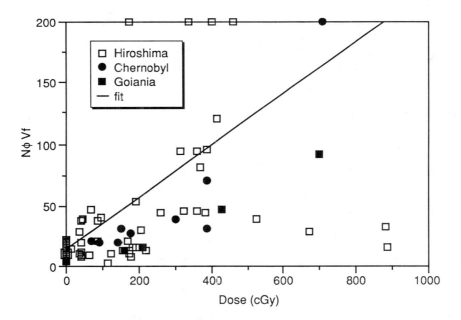

Fig. 4. GPA variant frequencies in individuals exposed to whole-body ionizing radiation. Assay results in survivors of the atomic bombing of Hiroshima, the Chernobyl nuclear reactor accident, and an accidental exposure to a ^{137}Cs source in Goiania, Brazil.

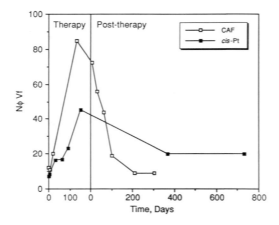

Fig. 5. GPA variant frequencies in cancer patients undergoing chemotherapy. Assay results on patients before and after chemotherapy with two chemical regimens: CAF (cyclophosphamide, adriamycin, 5-fluorouracil) and *cis*-Pt (*cis*-platinum or carboplatinum, etoposide).

or no persistent mutagenic effects in the stem cells themselves. Alternatively, preliminary data indicates that treatment with *cis*-platinum(II) induces a lesser initial response, but variant frequencies remain significantly higher than pretherapy levels years after treatment. Thus, a significant fraction of the genetic damage induced by this agent appears to be fixed in bone marrow stem cells and stably persists. Since the mutagenic agents used in chemotherapy deliver a dispersed sublethal dose to the erythropoietic cell population, the GPA assay is ideally suited to quantitate the effects of these exposures.

Two of our studies have now provided evidence for an association between elevated risk of cancer and radiation-induced increases in GPA variant frequencies. The most compelling data comes from the study of A-bomb survivors (Fig. 4), which show dose-dependent increases in both GPA variant cell frequency [66,67] and leukemia mortality, as well as cancers of the esophagus, stomach, colon, lung, breast, ovary, urinary bladder, and central nervous system, and multiple myeloma

[70–72]. In addition, a recent examination of several women treated in the 1940s with intrauterine radium implants for "benign gynecologic disorders" demonstrated elevated levels of loss and duplication variants (Fig. 6). The location of the irradiation is particularly important, since about 30% of total bone marrow cells are present in the pelvic girdle. We estimate that the bone marrow in this region sustained an exposure of about 180 cGy over 24 h. This group of women has subsequently been shown to be at increased risk for leukemia, incurring a twofold increase in leukemia mortality over lifetime, including an eightfold increase in the 2–5 year period following treatment [73].

LIMITATIONS OF PREDICTIVE APPLICATION OF THE GPA ASSAY

The GPA assay, as it is presently performed, quantitates the presence of erythrocytes with aberrant phenotypes as a frequency per total erythrocyte population. In order to predict how often these segregation events occur and, therefore, predict when a recurrence of childhood

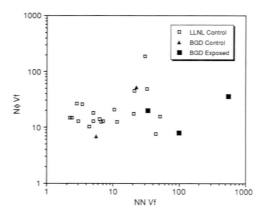

Fig. 6. GPA variant frequencies in individuals following radiotherapy for benign gynecological disorders. Included for reference are data from a subset of LLNL women retirees over 65 years of age and two elderly control women from the same geographic area as the treated individuals.

cancer might occur, this frequency must be converted to a rate, by quantitating the number of events per cell generation. This is a difficult task in the hematopoietic system, where the total erythrocyte population turns over every 120 days and an unknown number of stem cells are contributing to the population at any one time [24]. Moreover, similar developmental data must be available concerning the tissue(s) at risk for secondary neoplasia. Some evidence that the tissue of origin modulates the kinetics of onset of genetically predisposed neoplasia comes from the retinoblastoma locus, where "familial" cases often manifest retinal tumors in the first year of life, but having survived this period may not suffer the related osteosarcoma or soft tissue sarcoma for decades [47–54].

Cell growth kinetics may also potentially affect tissue susceptibility to cancer in a more straightforward manner. Several of the allele loss and loss and duplication mechanisms shown in Figure 2 are either exclusively mitotic events or may be influenced by the duration and fidelity of cell division and mitosis. Thus, recombinational events such as somatic crossover and gene conversion, as well as some translocations, inversions, and deletions, require the chromosome pairing and chromatin manipulating enzymes present during the DNA synthesis phase of cell division in order to occur. Likewise, missegregation events, such as the single aberrant disjunction or series of two nondisjunctions that we have postulated as contributing to the loss and duplication class of variants, must occur during mitosis, since it is otherwise difficult to account for the generation of a second intact copy of the chromosome carrying the variant allele. While chromosome loss can occur randomly at any phase of the cell cycle, there is certainly a contribution from simple nondisjunction at mitosis. Similarly, while gene inactivation may also occur at

any time, the one known mechanism of inactivation, DNA methylation, requires the action of a methylase enzyme. There are no known de novo methylases in adult mammalian cells, suggesting that aberrant gene inactivation is a consequence of misdirected action of the maintenance methylase that functions to restore complete methylation at a hemimethylated CG site after mitosis [74]. Thus, the differential cell growth kinetics of our target tissue, hematopoetic bone marrow stem cells, and the tissue(s) at risk for cancer may not only affect the relative number of cell generations cells have undergone, but since many of these mutational and segregational events are associated with mitosis itself, they may affect the frequencies of these events as well.

Another caveat to the direct application of GPA variant frequencies to recurrence estimates involves the so-called "position effect." The chromosomal position of a recessive oncogene relative to the centromere will certainly affect the frequency of the cross-over events involved in both mitotic recombination and gene conversion. In addition, position effects refer to the gene complement flanking the gene of interest. The potentially deleterious or lethal effects of reduction to monosomy or even nullisomy of these flanking markers help determine whether a cell having undergone segregation simply dies, is outcompeted by its neighbors, or succumbs to neoplasia. The GPA locus itself, to the best of our knowledge, acts as a neutral reporter in this assay, since there are no known advantages associated with either allele. Indeed, GPA-null individuals have been reported who manifest no deleterious effects [30,35]. Such neutrality would not be expected for all genes, however, especially those that can affect tumorigenicity. The effects of segregational events on adjoining loci would therefore be expected to affect the frequency and mechanisms of mutational and segregational events detectable or allowable at any locus. This limitation should become obvious in comparisons between the GPA assay and the HPRT mutation assay, since the X chromosome is functionally hemizygous in humans. Finally, position effects may occur that are the result of preexisting chromosomal lesions, such as fragile sites and small inversions, which are known to affect chromosome breakage, deletion, and recombination [75–78].

There are also predictive limitations associated with the target cells for our assay, the erythropoietic stem cells of the bone marrow. For example, our assay does not manifest elevated variant frequencies in individuals afflicted with xeroderma pigmentosum, presumably because their intolerance to UV irradiation is inconsequential to cells sequestered in the bone marrow. It is therefore important to develop complementary assays to the GPA assay, using markers at different sites in the genome and affecting different, if possible multiple, target tissues. Only then can the importance of these effects be measured and appropriate predictions of secondary tumors be made with confidence.

Finally, it is clear that few cancers will have as simple a genetic basis as retinoblastoma. Indeed, the difference in ages of onset between retinoblastoma and osteosarcoma might be explained not by tissue-type differences but by the requirement for an additional reduction to homozygosity at a second locus in the latter cancer [55]. Certainly, cancers with far more complicated requirements, including contributions from both known classes of oncogene, are now being described [56], and the recurrence kinetics for these types of cancer are sure to be complex. Indeed, when multiple events are required for oncogenesis, no simple mutational and/or segregational model or assay will be able to give more than a general impression of the frequency of possible recurrence.

CONCLUSIONS

The GPA assay, by measuring the frequency of molecular events that give rise to cancer, shows potential as a means of screening a population in order to determine those individuals at particular risk for neoplasia. Since an unusually high frequency of fixed mutational or segregational events should be deleterious, such individuals should be rare. Thus, cancer incidence should be associated generally with the background frequency of GPA variants in a population. Variant frequencies can, however, be affected by environmental or occupational exposure to mutagens, and probably clastogens as well, with some of the most significant exposures associated with cancer treatment. Thus, in a putative prospective study of the correlation of GPA variant frequencies with carcinogenesis, most individuals in the study population should have background frequencies of GPA variants, and cancer should arise in these individuals at rates consistent with current epidemiological data. A small number of individuals should manifest unusually high GPA variant frequencies, and this population should be at higher risk for cancers of the sporadic type. Individuals in the population who are exposed to circumstances such as cancer treatment, which increase their GPA variant frequencies in either the short term or in the long term, should also be at increased cancer risk. Hidden among the large "normal" population should be those rare individuals who carry a high risk of cancer because of predisposition at a particular locus, such as retinoblastoma. Cancer incidence in these individuals, both primary neoplasia and recurrence, should again be consistent with epidemiological studies and be associated with normal GPA variant frequencies. An individual unfortunate enough to have both a specific cancer predisposition and high GPA variant frequencies would be at even higher risk for recurrence. Moreover, cancer recurrence is probably rarely associated with either genetic predisposition or mutagenic induction alone, but by both mechanisms acting synergistically [79]. The cancer-prone syndromes were not discovered necessarily because of their higher de novo frequency of mutagenic or segregational events (indeed, XP patients do not show such a characteristic), but by their increased sensitivity to mutagen exposure [60]. Thus, the manner of treatment of a primary cancer in an individual with high GPA variant frequencies should reflect their increased de novo cancer risk, and possibly their increased sensitivity to mutagens.

Finally, we have taken great pains in this chapter to dissociate the GPA assay itself from cancer incidence or predisposition. There is no evidence that reduction to homozygosity of the GPA locus itself is associated with oncogenesis, and, indeed, it is hard to imagine how gene-specific events at this locus might affect the susceptibility of an individual to cancer. We are only now beginning to search for all the potential recessive oncogenes present in the human genome, however, and if our experience with proto-oncogenes is any guide, a large number of these genes will be found, spread randomly throughout the genome. It should not be surprising, therefore, that the recessive oncogene responsible for primary hepatocellular carcinoma has recently been mapped to human chromosome 4 [80]. Thus, the chromosomal events that we measure in the erythropoetic lineage with the GPA assay, which result in no deleterious effects that we are aware of, may actually contribute directly to neoplasia when they occur in the liver.

ACKNOWLEDGMENTS

The authors gratefully acknowledge all the participating physicians who contributed to these investigations, Barbara A. Nisbet and Ann E. Gorvad for excellent technical assistance, and Barbara R. DuPont, Ph.D. and Jean J. Latimer, Ph.D. for critical reading of the manuscript. This work was performed under the auspices of the U.S. Department of Energy at the Lawrence Livermore National Laboratory under contract number W-7405-ENG-48, with support from the U.S. EPA (grant R-811819), the U.S. NIEHS (interagency agreement NIH-ES-83-14), and the U.S. NIH (grant CA 48518).

REFERENCES

1. Langlois RG, Bigbee WL, Jensen RH: Measurements of the frequency of human erythrocytes with gene expression loss phenotypes at the glycophorin A locus. Hum Genet 74:353–362, 1986.
2. Langlois RG, Nisbet BA, Bigbee WL, Ridinger DN, Jensen RH: An improved flow cytometric assay for somatic mutations at the glycophorin A locus in humans. Cytometry 11:513–521, 1990.
3. Maron DM, Ames BN: Revised methods for the Salmonella mutagenicity test. Mut Res 113:173–215, 1983.
4. Thompson LH, Baker RM: Isolation of mutants of cultured mammalian cells. In Prescott MD (ed): Methods in Cell Biology (Vol VI). New York: Academic Press, 1973, pp 209–281.
5. Fox M, Rossiter BJF, Brennand J: Different mechanisms of reversion of HPRT-deficient V79 Chinese hamster cells. Mutagenesis 3:15–21, 1988.
6. Fuscoe JC, Fenwick RG, Ledbetter DH, Caskey CT: Deletion and amplification of the HGPRT locus in Chinese hamster cells. Mol Cell Biol 3:1086–1096, 1983.
7. Fenwick RG, Fuscoe JC, Caskey CT: Amplification versus mutation as a mechanism for reversion of a HGPRT mutation. Somat Cell Genet 10:71–84, 1984.
8. Gossler A, Joyner AL, Rossant J, Skarnes WC: Mouse embryonic stem cells and reporter constructs to detect developmentally regulated genes. Science 244:463–465, 1989.
9. Shih C, Shilo B, Goldfarb M, Dannenberg A, Weinberg R: Passage of phenotypes of chemically transformed cells via transfection of DNA and chromatin. Proc Natl Acad Sci USA 76:5714–5718, 1979.
10. Krontiris TG, Cooper GM: Transforming activity of human tumor DNAs. Proc Natl Acad Sci USA 78:1181–1184, 1981.

11. Fasano O, Birnbaum D, Edlund L, Fogh J, Wigler M: New human transforming genes detected by a tumorigenicity assay. Mol Cell Biol 4:1695–1705, 1984.

12. Beck TW, Huleihel M, Gunnell M, Bonner TI, Rapp UR: The complete coding sequence of the human A-*raf*-1 oncogene and transforming activity of a human A-*raf* carrying retrovirus. Nucleic Acids Res 15:595–609, 1987.

13. Eva A, Vecchio G, Diamond M, Tronick SR, Ron D, Cooper GM, Aaronson SA: Independently activated *dbl* oncogenes exhibit similar yet distinct structural alterations. Oncogene 1:355–360, 1987.

14. Noguchi T, Galland F, Batoz M, Mattei M-G, Birnbaum D: Activation of a *mcf.2* oncogene by deletion of amino-terminal coding sequences. Oncogene 6:709–715, 1988.

15. Murnane JP, Yezzi MJ: Association of high rate of recombination with amplification of dominant selectable gene in human cells. Somat Cell Mol Genet 14:273–286, 1988.

16. Biedler JL, Spengler BA: Metaphase chromosome anomaly: Association with drug resistance and cell-specific products. Science 191:185–187, 1976.

17. Siminovitch L: Mechanisms of genetic variation in Chinese hamster ovary cells. In Gottesman MM (ed): Molecular Cell Genetics. New York: Wiley, 1985, pp 869–879.

18. Pool BL, Yalkinoglu AO, Klein P, Schlehofer JR: DNA amplification in genetic toxicology. Mutat Res 213:61–72, 1989.

19. Heilbronn R, zur Hausen H: A subset of herpes simplex virus replication genes induces DNA amplification within the host cell genome. J Virol 63:3683–3692, 1989.

20. Cavolina P, Agnese C, Maddalena A, Sciandrello G, Di Leonardo A: Induction of CAD gene amplification by restriction endonucleases in V79.B7 Chinese hamster cells. Mutat Res 225:61–64, 1989.

21. Endow SA, Atwood KC: Magnification: Gene amplification by an inducible system of sister chromosome exchange. Trends Genet 4:348–351, 1988.

22. Albertini RJ, Castle KL, Borcherding WR: T-cell cloning to detect the mutant 6-thioguanine-resistant lymphocytes present in human peripheral blood. Proc Natl Acad Sci USA 79:6617–6621, 1982.

23. Albertini RJ, O'Neill JP, Nicklas JA, Recio L, Skopek TR: *hprt* mutations in vivo in human T-lymphocytes: Frequencies, spectra and clonality. Prog Clin Biol Res 340C: 15–24, 1990.

24. Loken MR, Shah VO, Dattilio KL, Civin CI: Flow cytometric analysis of human bone marrow: I. Normal erythroid development. Blood 69:255–263, 1987.

25. Siebert PD, Fukuda M: Human glycophorin A and B are encoded by separate, single copy genes coordinately regulated by a tumor-promoting phorbol ester. J Biol Chem 261: 12433–12436, 1986.

26. Shows TB, McAlpine PJ: The 1981 catalogue of assigned human genetic markers and report of the nomenclature committee. Cytogenet Cell Genet 32:221–245, 1982.

27. Rahuel C, London J, d'Auriol L, Mattei M-G, Tournamille C, Skrzynia C, Lebouc Y, Galibert F, Cartron J-P: Characterization of cDNA clones for human glycophorin A. Use for gene localization and for analysis of normal of glycophorin-A-deficient (Finnish type) genomic DNA. Eur J Biochem 172:147–153, 1988.

28. Kudo S, Fukuda M: Structural organization of glycophorin A and B genes: Glycophorin B gene evolved by homologous recombination at Alu repeat sequences. Proc Natl Acad Sci USA 86:4619–4623, 1989.

29. Race RR, Sanger R: Blood Groups in Man, 6th ed. Oxford: Blackwell Press, 1975, pp 92–138.

30. Furthmayer H: Structural comparison of glycophorins and immunochemical analysis of genetic variants. Nature 271:519–524, 1978.

31. Prohaska R, Koerner TAW Jr, Armitage IM, Furthmayer H: Chemical and carbon-13 nuclear magnetic resonance studies of the blood group M and N active sialoglycopeptides from glycophorin A. J Biol Chem 256:5781–5791, 1981.

32. Siebert PD, Fukuda M: Isolation and characterization of human glycophorin A cDNA clones by a synthetic oligonucleotide approach: Nucleotide sequence and mRNA structure. Proc Natl Acad Sci USA 83:1665–1669, 1986.

33. Siebert PD, Fukuda M: Molecular cloning of a human glycophorin B cDNA: Nucleotide sequence and genomic relationship to glycophorin A. Proc Natl Acad Sci USA 84:6735–6739, 1987.

34. Tate CG, Tanner CG: Isolation of cDNA clones for human erythrocyte membrane sialoglycoproteins α and δ. Biochem J 254:743–750, 1988.

35. Anstee DJ: Blood group MNSs-active sialoglycoproteins of the human erythrocyte membrane. In Sandler SG, Nusbacher J, Schanfield MS (eds): Immunobiology of the Erythrocyte. New York: Alan R. Liss, 1980, pp 67–98.

36. Pious D, Soderland C: HLA variants of cultured lymphoid cells: Evidence for mutational origin and estimation of mutation rate. Science 197:769–771, 1977.

37. Pious D, Soderland C, Gladstone P: Induction

of HLA mutations by chemical mutagens in human lymphoid cells. Immunogenetics 4:437–448, 1977.

38. Kavathas P, Bach FH, DeMars R: Gamma ray-induced loss of expression of HLA and glyoxalase I alleles in lymphoblastoid cells. Proc Natl Acad Sci USA 77:4251–4255, 1980.

39. Waldren C, Jones C, Puck TT: Measurement of mutagenesis in mammalian cells. Proc Natl Acad Sci USA 76:1358–1362, 1979.

40. Waldren C, Martin J, Sutherland J, Cram S: Use of somatic cell hybrids for quantitation of mutagenesis: Reduction in background mutants by fluorescence-activated cell sorting (FACS). Cytometry 5:584–588, 1984.

41. Waldren C, Jones C: Chromosome loss and damage as measured by biological markers. In Richmond CR, Walsh PJ, Copenhaver ED (eds): Health Risk Analysis: Proceedings of the Third Life Sciences Symposium. Philadelphia: The Franklin Institute Press, 1981, pp 333–344.

42. Turner DR, Morley AA, Haliandros M, Kutlaca R, Sanderson BJ: In vivo somatic mutations in human lymphocytes frequently result from major gene alterations. Nature 315:343–345, 1985.

43. Turner DR, Grist SA, Janatipour M, Morley AA: Mutations in human lymphocytes commonly involve gene duplication and resemble those seen in cancer cells. Proc Natl Acad Sci USA 85:3189–3192, 1988.

44. Janatipour M, Trainor KJ, Kutlaca R, Bennett G, Hay J, Turner DR, Morley AA: Mutations in human lymphocytes studied by an HLA selection system. Mutat Res 198:221–226, 1988.

45. McCarron MA, Kutlaca A, Morley AA: The HLA-A mutation assay: Improved technique and normal results. Mutat Res 225:189–193, 1989.

46. Hungerford J, Kingston J, Plowman N: Orbital recurrence of retinoblastoma. Ophthalmic Pediatr Genet 8:63–68, 1987.

47. DerKinderin DJ, Koten JW, Nagelkerke NJ, Tan KE, Beemer FA, Den Otter W: Non-ocular cancer in patients with hereditary retinoblastoma and their relatives. Int J Cancer 41:499–504, 1988.

48. Lueder GT, Judisch F, O'Gorman TW: Second nonocular tumors in survivors of heritable retinoblastoma. Arch Ophthalmol 104:372–373, 1986.

49. Draper GJ, Sanders BM, Kingston JE: Second primary neoplasms in patients with retinoblastoma. Br J Cancer 53:661–671, 1986.

50. Mitchell C: Second malignant neoplasms in retinoblastoma. Fact and fiction. Ophthalmic Pediatr Genet 9:161–165, 1988.

51. Roarty JD, McLean IW, Zimmerman LE: Incidence of second neoplasms in patients with bilateral retinoblastoma. Ophthalmology 95:1583–1587, 1988.

52. Reissmann PT, Simon MA, Lee WH, Slamon DJ: Studies of the retinoblastoma gene in human sarcomas. Oncogene 4:839–843, 1989.

53. Hansen MF, Koufos A, Gallie BL, Phillips RA, Fodstad O, Brogger A, Gedde Dahl T, Cavenee WK: Osteosarcoma and retinoblastoma: A shared chromosomal mechanism revealing recessive predisposition. Proc Natl Acad Sci USA 82:6216–6220, 1985.

54. Weichselbaum RR, Beckett M, Diamond A: Some retinoblastomas, osteosarcomas, and soft tissue sarcomas may share a common etiology. Proc Natl Acad Sci USA 85:2106–2109, 1988.

55. Toguchida J, Ishizaki K, Nakamura Y, Sasaki MS, Ikenaga M, Kato M, Sugimoto M, Kotoura Y, Yamamuro T: Assignment of common allele loss in osteosarcoma to the subregion 17p13. Cancer Res 49:6247–6251, 1989.

56. Vogelstein B, Fearon ER, Hamilton SR, Kern SE, Preisinger AC, Leppert M, Nakamura Y, White R, Smits AM, Bos JL: Genetic alterations during colorectal-tumor development. N Engl J Med 319:525–532, 1988.

57. Grant SG, Bigbee WL, Langlois RG, Jensen RH: Allele loss at the human GPA locus: A model for recessive oncogenesis (Abstr). Clin Biotech 1:66, 1989.

58. Bigbee WL, Wyrobek AW, Langlois RG, Jensen RH, Everson RB: The effect of chemotherapy on the in vivo frequency of glycophorin A "null" variant erythrocytes. Mutat Res 240:165–176, 1990.

59. Manchester DK, Grant SG, Langlois RG, Jensen RH, Bigbee WL: Occurrence of glycophorin A phenotypic variants in human umbilical cord blood (Abstr). Am J Hum Genet 47(suppl): A139.

60. German J: Patterns of neoplasia associated with the chromosome-breakage syndromes. In German J (ed): Chromosome Mutation and Neoplasia. New York: Alan R. Liss, 1983, pp 97–134.

61. Bigbee WL, Langlois RG, Swift M, Jensen RH: Evidence for an elevated frequency of in vivo somatic cell mutations in ataxia telangiectasia. Am J Hum Genet 44:402–408, 1989.

62. Langlois RG, Bigbee WL, Jensen RH, German J: Evidence for increased in vivo mutation and somatic recombination in Bloom's syndrome. Proc Natl Acad Sci USA 86:670–674, 1989.

63. Kyoizumi S, Nakamura N, Takebe H, Tatsumi K, German J, Akiyama M: Frequency of variant erythrocytes at the glycophorin-A locus in two Bloom's syndrome patients. Mutat Res 214:215–222, 1989.

64. Langlois RG, Bigbee WL, Jensen RH: The glycophorin A assay for somatic cell mutations in humans. Prog Clin Biol Res 340C:47–56, 1990.

65. Albertini RJ, DeMars R: Mosaicism of peripheral blood lymphocyte populations in females heterozygous for the Lesch–Nyhan syndrome. Biochem Genet 11:397–411, 1974.

66. Langlois RG, Bigbee WL, Kyoizumi S, Nakamura N, Bean MA, Akiyama M, Jensen RH: Evidence for increased somatic cell mutations at the glycophorin A locus in atomic bomb survivors. Science 236:445–448, 1987.

67. Kyoizumi S, Nakamura N, Hakoda M, Awa AA, Bean MA, Jensen RH, Akiyama M: Detection of somatic mutations at the glycophorin A locus in erythrocytes of atomic bomb survivors using a single beam flow sorter. Cancer Res 49:581–588, 1989.

68. Straume T, Langlois RG, Lucas J, Jensen RH, Bigbee WL, Ramalho AT, Brandao-Mello CE: Novel biodosimetry methods applied to the victims of the Goiania accident. Health Phys 60:71–76.

69. Mendelsohn ML: New approaches for biological monitoring of radiation workers. Health Phys 59:23–28, 1990.

70. Monzen T, Wakabayashi T: Tumor and tissue registries in Hiroshima and Nagasaki. In Shigematsu I, Kagan A (eds): Cancer in Atomic Bomb Survivors. New York: Plenum Press, 1986, pp 29–40.

71. Preston DL, Pierce DA: The effect of changes in dosimetry on cancer mortality risk estimates in the atomic bomb survivors. Radiat Res 114:437–466, 1988.

72. Shimizu Y, Kato H, Schull WJ: Life span study report 11 part 2. Cancer mortality in the years 1950–85 based on the recently revised doses (DS86). Radiation Effects Research Foundation Technical Report 5, 1988.

73. Inskip PD, Monson RR, Wagoner JK, Stovall M, Davis FG, Kleinerman RA, Boice JD Jr: Leukemia following radiotherapy for uterine bleeding. Radiat Res 122:107–119, 1990.

74. Jones PA, Taylor SM: Hemimethylated duplex DNAs prepared from 5-azacytidine-treated cells. Nucleic Acids Res 9:2933–2947, 1981.

75. Glover TW, Stein CK: Chromosome breakage and recombination at fragile sites. Am J Hum Genet 43:265–273, 1988.

76. Ronen A: Interchromosomal effects on somatic recombination in *Drosophila melanogaster.* Genetics 50:649–658, 1964.

77. Kafer E: Meiotic and mitotic recombination in *Aspergillus* and its chromosomal aberrations. Adv Genet 19:33–131, 1977.

78. Silver LM: Mouse t haplotypes: A tale of tails and a misunderstood selfish chromosome. Curr Top Microbiol Immunol 137:64–69, 1988.

79. Schwarz MB, Burgess LP, Fee WE, Donaldson SS: Postirradiation sarcoma in retinoblastoma. Induction or predisposition? Arch Otolaryngol Head Neck Surg 114:640–644, 1988.

80. Buetow HK, Murray JC, Israel JL, London WT, Smith M, Kew M, Blanquet V, Brechot C, Redeker A, Govindarajah S: Loss of heterozygosity suggests tumor suppressor gene responsible for primary hepatocellular carcinoma. Proc Natl Acad Sci USA 86:8852–8856, 1989.

18

How Am I Different? Perspectives of Childhood Cancer Survivors on Change and Growth

Mark A. Chesler, Ph.D., Margaret Weigers, M.A., and Timothy Lawther, B.A.

Advances in the diagnosis and treatment of childhood cancer have greatly extended the life spans of youngsters diagnosed with various forms of this disease. For many, it has led to the real possibility of a long-term cure. With these advances has come a corollary shift in the nature of psychosocial research on the life experiences and outlooks of children with cancer. Early work focusing on their adaptation to a terminal illness and anticipation of death has given way, over time, to a focus on the processes of coping with a chronic and serious illness, one with an increasing chance of long-term survival. Most recently, some research has begun to focus on the survivors themselves, attempting to understand the ways these young people dealt with their diagnosis and treatment, how they approach their present and future life experiences, and what may (or may not) distinguish them from other young people without a history of cancer.

Since the prospect of long-term survival from childhood cancer is still a relatively recent phenomenon, few large-scale and systematic studies have been undertaken. Those that have examined this population, and the issues they experience, have done so from a variety of approaches: some with small samples and a clinical psychological (perhaps psychopathological) perspective and others with a large sample and a social adaptational (or normal/healthy coping) perspective; some with standardized psychometric measures and others with uniquely devised questions or instruments; some with young people all being treated at the same institution, and others with a population drawn from several centers in a given geographical area; some with survivors of one type of childhood cancer, and others with young people with different types of cancer; some conducted (and controlled) by a treatment institution and others conducted outside of these centers; some with random (or sibling) control groups and others without such comparisons; some with a desire to test or impose theories generated in advance and others with a desire to describe and conceptualize the life experiences and perspectives of the young people studied; some attempting to speak for this population, and others seeking to discover and reflect the voices of this population themselves. With a (sub)field of inquiry in such an early stage of development, this variety is to be expected, perhaps even to be cherished.

One item in contention in the studies that have been done involves the very definition of a "survivor." In truth, any young person found to have cancer is (and should be treated as) a survivor from the

Late Effects of Treatment for Childhood Cancer, pages 151–158 © 1992 Wiley-Liss, Inc.

moment of diagnosis—he/she is surviving immediately. This orientation suggests that survival be considered a process rather than a state of being. However, most research restricts the term to young people with a cancer history who are successfully off treatment, in remission for several years, as we do in this chapter.

Our own research and action projects stem from a decade of psychosocial work. In addition to conducting research on these issues, we have been involved in education and peer counseling activities with families, organizing self-help groups and training group leaders, and consulting with medical care providers. We have also attempted to influence the voluntary and public agencies that make policy and delivery of psychosocial and community services to these groups, families, and individuals.

METHODS

The Candlelighters' Childhood Cancer Foundation (CCCF) recently sponsored a study of the experiences and issues faced by long-term survivors of childhood cancer. A four-page questionnaire was distributed in the foundation's Youth Newsletter (CCCF, 1988), requesting young people with cancer who were over 14 years of age and off all treatment to respond. Almost 300 long-term survivors of childhood cancer between the ages of 14 and 29 responded from all parts of the United States. In addition to these questionnaires, several group discussions (focus groups) were held with small groups of long-term survivors in different parts of the nation.

One limitation of this procedure is that we have almost no knowledge of who or how many young people did not respond to the questionnaire, or why they did not choose to do so. Generalizations must be made cautiously without such response rate data, and without good sample control. On the other hand, the responses to

the questionnaire and group interviews are so rich and detailed that they provide a level of information and meaning that often offers a suitable basis for broader interpretation. Finally, we distributed a slightly altered version of the questionnaire to a sample of high school and college age young people without a history of childhood cancer, and responses from this population provide us with vital comparisons with the long-term survivor population on many variables.

One of the closed-ended questions asked on the long-term survivor questionnaire was whether informants agreed or disagreed that "Having cancer has made me different from others of my age." In addition, informants were asked to indicate, in answer to an open-ended question, "In what ways are you different from other young people your age?" This chapter presents preliminary results of our analyses of the answers to these questions and explores the relationship between these items and other demographic, medical status, and attitudinal variables.

Our research staff combines the expertise of trained social scientists and people directly involved with the experience of childhood cancer. The senior staff member is a parent of a long-term survivor of childhood cancer, and two younger staff members are themselves long-term survivors. All these and other colleagues are trained in techniques of social science inquiry. In addition to this research staff, the collaboration between the University of Michigan and the CCCF generates a constant dialogue between insiders and outsiders, between more objective and more subjective inquiry modes, and among survivors and their parents and scholars. Our action–research approach means that we are constantly designing studies with members of the population under inquiry, sharing preliminary results with them (in attempts at "member verification"), and involving them in the design of service programs or policy changes based on the knowledge generated. It has been our experience that this participatory mode of inquiry has numerous benefits. Not the least of them is an increased ability to untangle the many knotty problems such as data gathering and interpretation of problems that are involved in research on sensitive and complex psychosocial matters, fraught as they are with subjective meaning and concern.

RESULTS

Forty-six percent of the long-term survivor informants "strongly agreed" that they were different from others their age, and 77% "agreed" with this closed-ended statement overall. On the open-ended question, 76% indicated that they felt different from their age peers: 13% said they were not different and 11% did not answer this question. Thus, the distribution of responses on the closed and open-ended items are quite comparable.

Of those young people who indicated, on the open-ended question, that they did feel differently from other young people their age, 69% mentioned differences that

were positive and 31% mentioned differences that were negative (Table 1). This is the first clear finding: most of the ways in which these survivors feel different from their peers are positive. The most frequent difference reported (30%), a positive one, was the survivors' feeling that they are more advanced or mature in their personality or psychological development than are their peers. Consider some of their statements:

I grew up faster. I value life a lot more. I'm a happy person being me and I don't need alcohol or drugs.

I strive hard in life. Chemotherapy was a hard struggle and I fought the battle and won. Therefore, I feel stronger than others mentally.

I think I grew up faster, although I didn't have a choice. My illness has allowed me to put things in perspective. Trivial things affect me less now (in school, grades, sports).

While these statements reflect a positive perspective, they are not naive or Pollyannish in tone. They convey a realistic sense of struggle and at least some of its specific effects.

A second common difference noted (18%), also a positive one, focused on an

TABLE 1. Long-Term Survivor Reports on How They Are Different From Other Young People

Differences	No.	(%)
Positive health differences	7	3
Positive developmental/personality differences	81	30
Positive social differences	5	2
Positive existential differences	49	18
No differences	34	13
Negative health/physical differences	43	16
Negative development/personality differences	11	4
Negative social differences	11	4
No answer	30	11
Total positive statements	142	52
Total negative statements	65	24
Total no response/no difference	64	24
Total responses	271	100/101

outlook on life in general—an "existential perspective." Many young people who are off-treatment indicated that they feel they know more about life and their purpose in life than do their peers.

I realize what is important in life and I don't take everything for granted. I want to live life to the fullest.

Having faced the idea of dying has made me look at life in a different way—to respect life and what I have each day.

I think the most important thing is—I live life for today because no one promised me tomorrow.

We each have our favorite existential perspective and outlook on the meaning of life; we each make decisions about what it means to have a meaningful life. These survivors' responses focus on finding meaning in everyday encounters and activities, and emphasizing them. At the same time, other comments indicate that this focus includes long-range planning for the future.

The third most common difference (16%) was a negative one—their physical health status and abilities. They often felt less healthy and less physically able than their peers who did not have a history of cancer.

I can't play contact sports and I have a central line.

I lack physical stamina.

I can't run that fast. I can't tie shoes that good. I can't remember that good.

Table 1 also lists some other categories in which survivors indicate differences between themselves and their peers. These include: positive health differences, positive social/relationship differences, negative personality/developmental differences, and negative social/relationship differences. While of interest, the numbers and percentages of responses in these categories are too small to warrant further discussion.

Characteristics of Survivors Who Feel Different

Several forms of analysis were used to compare those young people who indicated they felt different from their peers with those who did not, and those who reported positive differences, negative differences, or no difference.

Both gender and age distinguished informants. A significantly higher proportion of young women than men reported feeling different, as did older survivors compared with younger ones. Moreover, in both instances, the females and the older survivors reported more negative differences than did their male and younger counterparts. Perhaps women and older adolescents (or older young adults) are involved in a social environment that requires them to be more aware of their status and personal history, and that treats these histories as more important (and more negative).

Most of the medically relevant characteristics we assessed (diagnosis, time since diagnosis, and relapse) were not related to reports of difference. However, those survivors who reported having visible side-effects of their treatment (67% of the population) were somewhat more likely to report feeling different, and to report that these differences were positive. Indeed, other research has reported that it may be "easier" to adapt to an illness whose side-effects are visible (to oneself and others) than to one whose markers are invisible. Acknowledging differences, even "negative" ones, may reflect an element of realistic self-appraisal, and thus be a positive coping strategy and evidence of positive self-esteem. To the extent that a "visible" side-effect is undeniable, it may be easier to acknowledge and cope with than an invisible (internal, physical, or emotional) scar.

The potential relationship between acknowledged differences and positive self-esteem is not simple; facing differences squarely also may mean admitting to certain worries or concerns. Informants who reported feeling different from others also more often reported worries about a number of issues. The genetic consequences of therapy, their reproductive capacities, their medical futures, and their ability to maintain friendships with peers were prominent concerns. On the other hand, they did not report worrying more often about their general health, their looks, their finances, or having a relapse.

Informants who reported feeling different from others reported less open and honest relationships with the medical staff, and less support from their family members—parents, grandparents, and siblings. While multivariate analyses are yet to be undertaken with these data, the latter two findings may well be a function of the increased age of those who most often reported feeling different. Maturity itself may be associated with more complex and less naive interpersonal relationships, and therefore, with less open medical interactions and a decrease in family support.

Finally, those informants who felt different also reported a significantly greater desire to have access to psychological counseling services. There is no indication that this reflects impending psychopathology or severe disturbance. Rather, it appears to be part of a positive and assertive desire to deal realistically and openly with past and present stresses and to make use of potentially helpful psychosocial resources. Many survivors also reported a desire for more information about "late-effects," and assistance in gaining health and life insurance. They also wanted help in finding oncologically sensitive physicians when they leave their family homes and clinics of original treatment for advanced educational or employment opportunities.

Informants who reported positive differences or negative differences were not distinguished from one another as strongly or as systematically as they both were from informants who reported not feeling different. Thus, the recognition and public acknowledgment of difference may be the critical factor in those who reported greater worries, poorer relationships with the staff, and less support. Perhaps less denial, or greater openness in confronting their situation, had led to greater openness in reporting and dealing with various concerns and dissatisfactions. Perhaps, too, the acknowledgment of difference accelerated recognition of other psychosocial needs and gaps in the support or service system.

This set of findings presents an image of young people in the midst of a struggle to identify themselves in their social world, given the nature of their unique medical experience. For the most part, the psychosocial outcomes of this struggle appear to be positive, but responders do not seem to overlook troublesome issues and needs.

How do we explain the prevalence of these positive feelings and positive self-assessments in this sample of long-term survivors? It could be that only those survivors who do feel positive and "upbeat" chose to respond to the questionnaire. Such a sample bias would so cloud the findings as to render the points moot. Perhaps sustained denial is at work. Indeed, some scholars and clinical practitioners have argued that denial of bad feelings and bad outcomes (and in this case, of negative differences) is a common and relatively healthy coping mechanism for children with cancer. Perhaps these young people are deliberately "lying" about their feelings or "falsifying" their outlooks in life for their own or our benefit. Some researches suggest that young people with cancer often hide their true distress or negative feelings from their physicians and parents, the better to protect themselves from intrusive procedures and their parents from further pain and burden.

The fact that the same young people who reported feeling positive and positively different also reported substantial worries about their futures alerts us to the complex and realistic struggle in which they feel they are engaged. This suggests that their responses are probably truthful. If they had denied all sense of worry and struggle, we might have less trust in the veracity of their positive responses.

Perhaps these young people wish to present themselves to the world in a positive and optimistic manner, regardless of the "true" mix of their feelings. By presenting themselves positively, they may help create a set of social expectations and interactions that are positive and accepting. They may, in this way, pro-actively counter negative expectations and cycles of pity, stigma, and prejudice. Moreover, by constructing a positive social environment and positive reactions from others, they can help reinforce a positive personal outlook. If they say they are doing well and can convince others that they are doing well, perhaps they can make and keep themselves well (psychologically, if not physically). The interaction between physical and mental health is too mysterious for us to dismiss this option out of hand.

It also is possible for us to take these reports at face value. Survivors of childhood cancer might just feel very positive about themselves, perhaps as an outgrowth of an inner transformation which we do not yet have access to or understand. We all search for meaning and confidence in our lives, and sometimes for benchmarks of our struggles and achievements with the forces of fate or other difficult tasks. These young people may feel they have engaged in, and mastered, just such a test, qualifying them for a special status. Thus, they may now root a part of their identity and sense of meaning in their achievement of victory in the struggle against cancer—surely a symbol of great danger,

mystery, and travail. Such a sense of accomplishment reasonably would lead to reports of lessons learned, confidence gained, positive outlooks, "specialness," and so on. Even while these young people acknowledge their physical and emotional scars, they often do sound and feel like victors rather than victims.

Others' Feelings of Difference

Feeling different and seeking individuation is common for people in our society, especially in the late adolescent age group from which these data were gathered. Just as common and potent, of course, is the desire to appear and feel normal and like others in one's peer network. In order to explore the universality of these issues further, we asked the comparison sample of high school and college age young people without a history of childhood cancer whether they felt different from others their age. Forty-four percent of this comparison sample agreed or strongly agreed on the closed-ended question that they were different, and 44% mentioned differences on the open-ended question. Seventy-nine percent of those informants who reported that they felt different mentioned positive differences. Those noted most often by this population included positive personality/developmental attributes (20%) and positive social skills/experiences (8%).

Comparisons Between Survivors' and Others' Feelings of Difference

In response to the closed-ended question, 77% of the survivor sample and 44% of the comparison sample agreed that they were different from others their age. In response to the open-ended question, 76% of the survivor sample and 44% of the comparison sample listed ways in which they were different from other young people. Although the survivor and comparison samples both reported "no difference" on the open-ended question in approximately equal proportions (13% vs 14%), the comparison sample most often did not answer this question. If we assume that nonresponse is a covert way of indication no difference, the total "no difference" response (*no difference* + *no response*) is much higher in the comparison sample (42 + 14 = 56%) than in the survivor sample (11 + 13 = 25%).

The survivor sample reported positive existential differences more often than did the comparison sample (18% vs 2%). They also more often expressed positive personality/developmental differences (30% vs 20%). In contrast, the survivor sample more often reported negative health differences (16% vs 3%) and somewhat less often positive social differences (2% vs 8%) than did the comparison sample.

The survivor sample had significantly more worries about their reproductive and genetic capacities, less worries about their looks and general health, more problems in schooling and in getting insurance, and more open and honest relationships with their physicians than did the comparison sample. Finally, survivors reported life habits that included significantly less exercise, less smoking, and less use of alcohol and recreational drugs than did the controls.

With the exception of the survivors' reports of less worry about general health issues, these findings all make immediate sense. Whether the report about general health is a straightforward example of denial or a reflection of more complex dynamics in the life experience or questionnaire responses of this population await further analysis. As noted previously, this report utilizes a preliminary analysis of a rich data set that will have to be studied further before these answers can be fully understood, if they can be at all. Planned studies include continuing discussions with long-term survivors of childhood cancer themselves. We want to know how they explain these results!

CONCLUSIONS

Young people who successfully complete treatment and enter the ranks of long-term survivors carry with them a sense of being different from others. The data resulting from our investigations make it clear that many of the distinctions from others that survivors detect are positive in nature, and reflect their feeling that they have been able to grow and develop positively from their medical experience.

But much of the data presented in this chapter clearly challenges some prior (and older) reports that predict a substantial incidence of depression and serious psychological problems in this population. The emphasis on positive differences is not without qualification. Survivors of childhood cancer also report a variety of worries and problems they experience in adapting to their world. These considerations suggest that informants are not presenting mindlessly or defensively positive messages but considered judgments about their present and future situations. At the very least, these outlooks are one major part of coping.

The struggle to serve the "truly cured child" requires careful attention to these issues of psychosocial adaptation and outlook. Psychosocial support services need to be designed and provided explicitly for this population. To design and provide services on the assumption of imminent psychopathology or maladjustment is not only wrong—given these data—but dangerous. It reiterates a cycle of negative expectations that may disable or discriminate against these survivors in their struggle to define and assert themselves.

Many long-term survivors wish to have the opportunity to share and compare their experiences and reactions with those of other young people with cancer and with medical and community groups. This would be a welcome addition to the resources at our disposal to educate the general public about childhood cancer. It would also help survivors achieve the psychological and social growth for which they clearly strive and deserve.

19

Enhancing the Adjustment of Long-Term Survivors: Early Findings of a School Intervention Study

M. List, Ph.D., C. Ritter-Sterr, M.S., R.N., and S. Lansky, M.D.

In pediatric oncology today, surviving cancer means overcoming not only the disease and its long-term physical effects, but also the psychological, social, and educational sequelae of the disease and its treatment. These psychosocial threats to optimal survival are numerous and include disruptions in peer relationships with resulting disturbances in social development, changes in family relationships and the risk of increased dependency between parent and child, changes in body image, and finally, disruptions in school attendance and performance.

The work described here focuses on one of these areas of concern, that is, school, particularly school attendance, as critical to the child's future development. This paper presents selected observations and intermediate results from two studies dealing with school performance and attendance. The first project is a pilot study of long-term survivors and the second is a large multiinstitutional intervention study currently in progress. The thrust of these projects is the development of intervention strategies aimed at prevention and early remediation of school problems with the goal of minimizing long-term difficulties.

STUDY 1—LONG-TERM SURVIVOR INTERVIEW

The objective of the first study was to examine the psychosocial adjustment of long-term survivors of childhood cancer, including an exploration of the impact of the disease at the time of diagnosis and treatment. The focus was on issues of school attendance, academic performance, and career achievement. Young adults who had cancer during adolescence and were at least five years from diagnosis were interviewed. The final sample consisted of 39 patients (49% male, 51% female) representing a range of pediatric malignancies (ALL, 15%; Hodgkin's disease, 46%; non-Hodgkin's lymphoma, 10%; osteogenic sarcoma, 15%). The mean age at the time of the interview was 23 years (range 16–33 years), the mean age at diagnosis was 13 years (range 11–16 years), and the time elapsed since the last treatment for cancer ranged from 15 months to 18 years (mean 7.1 years).

Questions about the immediate impact of the disease and its treatment confirmed the hypothesis that a diagnosis of cancer significantly disrupts a child's school life. Eighty-seven percent of the group reported disruptions in school attendance.

Late Effects of Treatment for Childhood Cancer, pages 159–164 © 1992 Wiley-Liss, Inc.

Over one-half of the sample (61%) indicated disruptions in peer relationships and decreases in participation in extracurricular activities (54%). Forty-six percent suggested that they had altered future academic plans and 38% reported changes in future career plans. Academic difficulties were described by 28% of the sample. Patients also described the distress and pain accompanying these disruptions. Many commented that they no longer "fit in" with their peers and felt isolated and alone.

These results are consistent with multiple reports of school-related problems. Children with cancer have been described as often having difficulty returning to school and maintaining attendance [1,2]. High rates of absenteeism have been reported with children missing an average of 21–45 days/year [3,4]. In one study average absenteeism rates in the year of diagnosis were as high as 53%, with hospitalization and clinic visits accounting for only 45% of days missed. Although absences declined to 14% by three years from diagnosis (vs 3% for national mean), only one-fourth of these were attributable to medical visits [5]. In addition, upon returning to school these children have been found to be less sociable [6], have trouble getting along with classmates [7], and face a range of general problems and unpleasant experiences [8,9].

The finding of such high rates of school disruption and absenteeism among children with cancer is an important observation with far-reaching implications. School is the center of a child's life and the primary setting of influence for both academic and social development. These functions are even more critical for the child who has cancer and already feels different. Being at school and participating in the normally shared intellectual and social activities of his/her peer group helps counteract the anxiety, depression, and isolation accompanying illness, while guiding psychosocial development. In addition, for a child who may have lasting physical impairments, the ability to achieve academically will be crucial.

Planning for all the school-related needs of the child with cancer is thus imperative. The necessary first step, however, is getting the child back to school. Children who do not return to school early may find it increasingly difficult to reintegrate at a later date. While these issues are being more widely recognized and addressed informally by some clinicians, systematic interventions have been minimal and generally unsuccessful. The majority of approaches described to date has focused on school personnel. Surveys have demonstrated that teachers [10,11] and nurses [12] need more information about childhood cancer and its implications for school. To meet these needs, workshops and educational presentations have been implemented, written materials distributed, and liasion between school and hospital personnel has been recommended [11,13–15]. However, although these programs are appreciated by school personnel, there has been little documentation that such efforts affect the child's attendance [15].

STUDY 2—BEHAVIORAL MANAGEMENT FOR SCHOOL ATTENDANCE

A follow-up intervention study focusing on school reentry was designed in response to these needs. This ongoing study is a prospective, multiinstitutional randomized trial testing the efficacy of a new intervention, a Behavioral Management Protocol for School Attendance. The protocol takes a preventive approach by intervening early, at the time of diagnosis, and relies on behavioral strategies implemented by the individual most likely to directly influence the child's behavior, that is, the parent.

The short-term objective of the study is to increase and maintain the school attendance of children with newly found cancer, and to minimize immediate discomfort and facilitate reintegration. The long-term goal is to minimize the social and academic difficulties of the long-term survivor. An equally important outcome of the study will be the acquisition of a data set that will include longitudinal information on attendance, achievement, and supporting medical and demographic variables in a sample of over 200 patients from across the country.

Subjects

All newly diagnosed school age (6–16 years) cancer patients with favorable prognosis are eligible for participation. These eligibility criteria were arrived at in collaboration with participating physicians and are designed to be inclusive, although most brain tumor and advanced disease patients are excluded.

Procedures/Assessment

Patients are randomly assigned to two groups: intervention and control, that is, no intervention. For all patients, assessments take place annually, beginning at intake, and include: demographic and disease-related data, records of school attendance (number of days absent) and achievement (grades), performance status (using Play Performance Scale) [16], and teacher and parent forms of the Child Behavior Checklist (social competence and behavior problems). In addition, attendance and achievement data are obtained for the year prior to diagnosis. Patients are followed for 2–5 years depending on point of study entry.

Intervention–Behavioral Management Protocol

The Behavioral Management Protocol is a school attendance intervention directed towards both prevention and early management of school attendance problems. It was designed to establish clearly the necessity of school attendance, to foster parental control and confidence, and to be practical and easily implemented across a variety of centers without the need for trained personnel.

The key to the Behavioral Management Protocol is the provision of a systemic step-by-step plan for use by the parent. It is presented simply, as a series of decision trees in diagram format. The protocol provides a framework for how and when to act by structuring preparation for return to school, discussing potential problems and solutions, and supplying illustrative scripts for responding to questions. The protocol provides parents with encouragement, helpful hints, and guidelines to facilitate decision-making. For example, to establish the expectation of a smooth return to school and to minimize missed schoolwork, the protocol instructs parents to set up early contact with the school and establish a system of receiving homework. Attempts are made to ease the child's anxieties and isolation by having the child maintain contact with a classmate when possible, suggesting ways that the child might explain his/her absence to the class (e.g., show and tell science projects) and providing sample responses to specific questions about hair loss, surgery, and so on. The protocol attempts to reassure the parent about the need for school even if the child is hesitant. It provides very specific directions for determining whether the child is sick enough to remain at home (e.g., criteria for illness predetermined by parent and physician) and provides step-by-step instructions for getting or taking, if necessary, a reluctant child to school.

In addition, parents of children in the intervention group complete monthly calendars on which they record their child's activity on any given day (e.g., in school, ill at home, in hospital, in clinic, vacation, or others). Parents maintain calendars for one year after diagnosis.

Results

To date, 180 children have been entered in the study and are currently being followed. The mean age of the group is 10 years and there are approximately equal numbers of boys and girls. The majority of the sample is white (86%), and the group represents a range of socioeconomic backgrounds and covers the full range of pediatric malignancies (leukemias, 51%; lymphomas, 26%; bone, 12%; others, 11%).

One-year follow-up data are available on 50 patients representing a follow-up rate of 85%. The majority of the sample received chemotherapy (98%). Approximately one-quarter received radiation therapy (26%), 10% had surgery, and 2% (one patient) had a bone marrow transplant. By the end of the first year, 12% of patients had relapsed and 12 patients had died. Over the year of diagnosis the average number of clinic visits per patient was 29 and average number of hospital admissions was five. At year one follow-up, the patients' disease status was described as follows: active treatment/disease free, 62%; active treatment/disease present, 12%; and no treatment/disease free, 26%.

Preliminary data summaries confirm that a cancer diagnosis significantly disrupts school attendance. Children in the study were missing very little school in the year before diagnosis (average of nine days/year). Not surprisingly, in the year of diagnosis the rate of absenteeism increased considerably with children missing close to 40 school days in the year (average 38). This pattern might be expected to change in the year after diagnosis but children were still missing an average of 37 school days, more than one day a week. These data were compiled from the total sample of children, that is, combining the intervention and no intervention groups. As adequate numbers of patients reach the first and second year follow-up assessment points, these calculations will be examined by group. An intervention effect is expected, that is, that there would be fewer days of school missed by children receiving the intervention as compared to children in the control group.

Data from a subset of the sample for whom parents completed monthly calendars enabled a closer examination of the pattern of school attendance across time. These data were organized in terms of the number of days the child was in school relative to the month of his/her diagnosis. In the months immediately following diagnosis, children attended very little school; for example, an average of four days in the month after diagnosis, up to seven days in the second month, and nine days in the third month. Days in school increased gradually over the next nine months but appeared to plateau at about 14 or 15 days a month out of a possible 20–23. Thus, by 12 months from diagnosis these children are still missing more than 1.25 days of school per week.

Some of the reasons for school absences are obvious and unavoidable. For example, illness resulting from the disease and/or treatment effects may necessitate hospitalization or otherwise preclude school attendance. Beyond these reasons, however, there are issues such as the parent's uncertainty and anxiety, and the child's dependency, fears, and embarrassment that may reinforce school absences. The current intervention addresses many of these potential interferences with the hope of both supporting the parent and increasing the child's attendance.

Summary and Future Directions

Data to date confirm that a cancer diagnosis leads to a significant disruption of school attendance. Preliminary analyses indicate no relationship between the rate of absenteeism and either diagnosis or personal demographics. Finally, while attendance does increase slowly during the months after diagnosis, rates only approach 75% by month 12. Further analyses of these data will address: a) group (intervention vs control) differences; b) the full range of possible predictive factors including sex, grade, size of school, and time of school year in which child was diagnosed; c) relationship between social competence, academic achievement, and attendance; and d) compliance with protocol as related to attendance data.

CONCLUSION

The many and varied problems of the long-term survivor are obviously multidetermined. The current work directly addresses one of these determinants—school. School is critical to both the immediate and long-term development of children, yet school reentry and attendance are problematic for the child with cancer. Despite reports of high rates of absenteeism, the few attempts to modify this behavior have been relatively unsuccessful. Thus the need for effective interventions to increase school attendance is imperative. The current study attempts to meet this need with the development and implementation of a behavioral intervention aimed at both prevention and early management of school-related problems. In addition, the study will develop a data set that will include valuable longitudinal information on attendance, achievement, and supporting medical and demographic variables on a sample of over 200 patients from across the country.

REFERENCES

1. Lansky SB, Lowman JT, Vats T, et al.: School phobia in children with malignant neoplasms. Am J Dis Child 129:42–46, 1975.
2. Stehbens JA, Kisker CT, Wilson BK: School behavior and attendance during the first year of treatment for childhood cancer. Psychol Sch 20:223–228, 1983.
3. Lansky SB, Cairns NU, Zwartes W: School attendance among children with cancer: A report from two centers. J Psychosoc Oncol 1:75–82, 1983.
4. Cairns NU, Klopovich P, Hearne E, Lansky SB: School attendance of children with cancer. J Sch Health 152–155, 1982.
5. Christy DM, Whitt JK, Lauria MM, McMillan CW, Wells RJ: Patterns of school re-entry for children with cancer (Abstract). Proc ASCO 7:A1054, 1988.
6. Noll RB, Bukoski WM, Rogosch FA, LeRoy S, Kulkarni R: Social interaction between children with cancer and their peers: Teacher ratings. J Pediatr Psychol 15:43–56, 1990.
7. Tebbi CK, Petrilli AS, Richards ME: Adjustment to amputation among adolescent oncology patients. Am J Pediatr Hematol Oncol 11:276–280, 1989.
8. Wasserman AL, Thompson EI, Williams JA, Fairclough DL: The psychological status of survivors of childhood/adolescent Hodgkin's disease. Am J Dis Child 141:626–631, 1987.
9. Mulhern RK, Wasserman AL, Friedman AG, Fairclough D: Social competence and behavioral adjustment of children who are long-term survivors of cancer. Pediatrics 83:18–25, 1989.
10. Deasy-Spinetta P, Spinetta JJ: The child with cancer in school: Teacher's appraisal. Am J Pediatr Hematol Oncol 2:89–94, 1980.
11. Fryer LL, Saylor CF, Finch AJ Jr, Smith KE: Helping the child with cancer: What school personnel want to know. Psychol Rep 65:563–566, 1989.
12. Moore IM, Triplett JL: Students with cancer: A school nursing perspective. Cancer Nurs 3:265–270, 1980.
13. Ross JW, Scarvalone SA: Facilitating the pediatric cancer patient's return to school. Social Work 27:256–261, 1982.
14. Ross JW: Resolving nonmedical obstacles to successful school reentry for children with cancer. J Sch Health 54:84–86, 1984.
15. Klopovich P, VanWezel G, Gaddy D, et al.:

School experiences of children with cancer: A collaborative nursing research study. Oncology Nursing Society Annual Meeting, 1982 (presented).

16. Lansky SB, List MA, Lansky LL, Ritter-Sterr C, Miller D: The measurement of performance in childhood cancer patients. Cancer 60:1651–1656, 1987.

20

Legal Remedies to Job and Insurance Discrimination Against Former Childhood Cancer Patients

Barbara Hoffman, J.D.

There are more than six million people alive in the United States today who have a history of cancer and face a working society that treats many of them differently solely because of their cancer histories [1]. Many of these persons are adult survivors of childhood cancer. Discrimination against qualified employees costs society billions of dollars in lost wages, lost productivity, and needless disability payments. In addition, irrational differential treatment cruelly isolates those who have struggled with cancer.

Paramount among the concerns of young cancer survivors is access to adequate, affordable health insurance. No state or federal law mandates universal health insurance. Whether termination from a plan, denial of benefits under a plan, or refusal to issue insurance violates a law is determined by two factors—the terms of the policy and the applicable law (federal and state).

CANCER-BASED EMPLOYMENT DISCRIMINATION

Scope of the Problem

Any type of job action may be affected by a cancer diagnosis: dismissal, failure to hire, demotion, denial of promotion, undesirable transfer, denial of benefits, and hostility in the workplace. Although some disparate treatments, such as blanket hiring bans against all individuals with a cancer history, are irrational and blatant, cancer-based discrimination is more often subtle and directed against an individual.

Approximately one in four survivors encounter cancer-related employment problems [2]. Cancer has a harsher impact on blue collar workers than on white collar workers. One author found that although 54% of white collar respondents described work problems that they attributed to cancer, 84% of the blue collar respondents identified such work problems [3].

Young adult survivors entering the job market for the first time are a rapidly growing population. In 1990, 1 of every 1,000 twenty-year olds was estimated to be a childhood cancer survivor [4]. Between 20% and 45% of them encountered cancer-related barriers to employment [5]. Younger cancer patients who are either employed or active in the labor market are more concerned than are older patients about revealing their cancer history in searching for another job [6].

One study comparing childhood cancer survivors with their siblings found that 80% of the male survivors were rejected from the military (as opposed to 18% of their siblings) and 32% were rejected from job opportunities (as opposed to 19% of

Late Effects of Treatment for Childhood Cancer, pages 165–170 © 1992 Wiley-Liss, Inc.

their siblings) [7]. Although female survivors faced disproportionate rejection from the military (75% as opposed to 13% for their siblings), the percentage of women rejected from employment was the same for survivors as for their siblings (19%).

Legal Remedies

Since the early 1970s, federal and state legislatures have passed a number of laws designed to prohibit employment discrimination based on medical conditions that do not affect an employee's qualifications. These laws vary widely in their scope and application to cancer-based discrimination.

Federal Laws

The Rehabilitation Act of 1973 [8] is the product of congressional recognition that employment barriers further the societal segregation of handicapped individuals [9]. Section 504 of the Act bans employment discrimination based on handicap by employers that receive federal financial assistance [10]. The Rehabilitation Act defines "handicapped individual" as

any person who 1) has a physical or mental impairment which substantially limits one or more of such person's major life activities; 2) has a record of such impairment; or 3) is regarded as having such an impairment [11].

The regulations to the Rehabilitation Act recognize that people with a cancer history often experience employment discrimination based on misconceptions about their illness long after they are fully recovered. The regulations provide that:

'has a record of such an impairment' means that an individual may be completely recovered from a previous physical or mental impairment. It is included because the attitude of employers, supervisors, and coworkers toward that previous impairment may result in an individual experiencing difficulty in securing,

retaining, or advancing in employment. The mentally restored, those who have had heart attacks, or *cancer* often experience such difficulty [12].

In 1988, the U.S. District Court for the Southern District of Texas became the first federal court to rule that the Rehabilitation Act of 1973 prohibits discrimination against an "otherwise qualified" person solely because of his cancer history [13]. After being successfully treated for cancer in 1981 as a young adult, Ray Ritchie applied for a position as a firefighter with the Houston Fire Department. The city rejected Ritchie's application solely because of his cancer history. The district court ruled that the city violated Ritchie's rights under the Rehabilitation Act by rejecting him solely because of his cancer history without making an individualized determination of his medical condition and qualifications [14]. In addition, the district court found that the city failed to establish that its medical standard is justified as a business necessity [15].

In addition to the Rehabilitation Act claim, the district court also ruled that the city violated Ritchie's right to the equal protection of the law guaranteed by the fourteenth amendment to the Constitution of the United States because its "medical standard excluding all cancer survivors on the basis of a supposed risk of harm to the cancer survivor is an arbitrary, unreasonable, and discriminatory classification" [16]. Ritchie was awarded backpay, benefits, and attorney fees [17].

The case of *Ritchie* leaves no doubt that the Rehabilitation Act prohibits cancer-based discrimination by a covered employer against a qualified individual with cancer. The primary limitation of the Rehabilitation Act is that it applies only to employers that receive federal financial assistance.

In mid-1990, Congress remedied this limitation with the passage of the Americans With Disabilities Act. The employment provisions of the Act, which are scheduled to take effect two years after President Bush signed the bill into law on July 26, 1990, prohibit employment discrimination based on disability by most private employers (those with at least 25 employees from 1992 to 1994, and 15 employees thereafter). Because the definition of a disabled person is modeled on the language of the Rehabilitation Act, cancer survivors, regardless of whether they are actually disabled, would be protected by the Americans With Disabilities Act.

State Rights

Until the Americans With Disabilities Act takes effect, cancer survivors who face discrimination, but are not covered by the Rehabilitation Act, must turn to state laws for relief. Every state has a law that regulates, to some extent, employment discrimination against people with disabilities. The application of these laws to cancer-based discrimination varies widely, however.

A few state laws explicitly prohibit discrimination against cancer survivors [18]. Other state statutes borrow language from Section 706 (7) (B) of the Rehabilitation Act to protect not only those who have a disability, but also those who are perceived to be disabled [19]. Because of a significant difference in the scope of state statutes, cancer-based discrimination clearly violates certain state laws (e.g., New York and Wisconsin) [20], may be illegal in other states (e.g., Texas and Illinois), and has never been adjudicated in the remaining states.

Although state discrimination laws differ substantially, they share one common element: Only _qualified_ workers are entitled to relief. An employee is qualified if he/she is able to perform in a reasonable manner the duties of the job in question. Most state, as well as federal, antidiscrimi-

nation laws appropriately balance the employee's right to equal job opportunities with the employer's right to consider only qualified applicants.

BARRIERS TO HEALTH INSURANCE

Scope of the Problem

Employment discrimination against cancer survivors affects survivors' wallets as well as their minds. The economic impact of cancer discrimination can be devastating. Most adults in the United States obtain health insurance through their employment [21]. Thus, denial of job opportunities means not only lost income but lost insurance benefits.

Until recently, inability to obtain an affordable insurance policy was the major insurance problem encountered by survivors. Approximately one in four cancer survivors are unable to obtain adequate health insurance [22]. Barriers to health insurance include refusal of new applications, policy cancellations or reductions, increased premiums, preexisting condition exclusions, and extended waiting periods.

Increasingly since the late 1980s, however, survivors have faced another insurance barrier: failure to be reimbursed for treatment deemed "experimental" by the insurance carrier and medically necessary by the oncologist. Most insurance policies do not cover "experimental" treatment. Insurance carriers have increasingly begun to label off-label chemotherapy and bone marrow transplantations as "experimental" to avoid large payments. A recent survey by the Association of Community Cancer Centers found that physicians now average four hours a week, and their staff 23 hours a week, seeking reimbursement for denied claims [23].

Legal Remedies

Neither states nor the federal government mandate a "legal right" to health insurance. Failure by an insurance company to comply with the terms of a policy is a question of state contract law (failure to pay a claim arguably covered by the policy may be a "breach of contract"). Access to health insurance is regulated primarily by state law, with the exception of two relatively new federal laws: COBRA (Consolidated Omnibus Reconciliation Act) and ERISA (Employee Retirement and Income Security Act).

Federal Laws

COBRA. COBRA [24] requires employers to offer group medical coverage to employees and their dependents who previously would have lost their group coverage because of individual circumstances. Public and private employers who have more than 20 employees are required to provide for continuation of insurance coverage in cases where an employee quits, is terminated, or works reduced hours. Coverage must extend to surviving, divorced, or separated spouses, and to dependent children.

Under COBRA, individuals who previously would have lost their insurance coverage because of a change in circumstances now may be provided continued group coverage for 18 months for themselves or 36 months for their spouses and dependents. Although they have to pay for the continued coverage, at rates that are usually more than group rates, the rates may not exceed 102% of the premium charged a similarly situated employee. Continuation of coverage must be offered regardless of any preexisting conditions, such as cancer. An employer found to have violated COBRA may lose his/her right to deduct health benefits from his/her federal taxes and may be required to provide an employee with benefits in accordance with the policy and the law.

ERISA. ERISA [25] may provide a remedy to an employee who has been denied full participation in an employee benefit plan because of a cancer history. Some employers fear that participation of a cancer survivor in a group medical plan will drain benefit funds or increase the employer's insurance premiums. A violation of ERISA may occur when an employer, upon learning of a worker's cancer history, dismisses that worker for the purpose of excluding him/her from a group health plan [26].

If the employer fires the employee for the purpose of cutting off that employee's benefits, regardless of whether the employee is considered handicapped under the statute, then the employer may be liable for a violation of ERISA. Employee benefit plans are defined widely, and include any plan with the purpose of providing "medical, surgical, or hospital care benefits, or benefits in the event of sickness, accident, disability, death, or unemployment." ERISA may be implicated if an employer encourages a person with a cancer history to retire as a "disabled" employee. "Disability" is usually defined in benefit plans as only the most debilitating conditions. Individuals with a cancer history often do not fit under such a definition and should not be compelled to so label themselves.

Under certain circumstances, ERISA may provide a cause of action to workers with a cancer history. ERISA covers both participants (employees) and beneficiaries (spouses and children). Thus, if the employee is fired because his/her child has cancer, ERISA may provide a cause of action. ERISA, however, is inapplicable to many instances of employment discrimination, including individuals who are denied a new job because of their medical status, employees who are subjected to differential treatment that does not impact on their benefits, and employees whose compensation does not include benefits.

State Laws

Every state has an insurance commission or department that enforces state regulation of insurance companies. The commission determines what types of policies must be offered and when rates may be raised. State regulations cover all aspects of health insurance, including rates, policy conditions (such as whether a policy must pay for screening mammograms), termination or reinstatement of coverage, and the scope of coverage and benefits. In 1990, New York and Michigan became the first states to require insurance policies that cover prescription drugs to pay for prescribed chemotherapy, regardless of whether the use is off-label.

Some states offer "high-risk pools" for the medically uninsurable. By June 1990, 25 states offered high-risk pools and many others had pending legislation. Although these laws differ in the amount of relief they provide, they share several common points.

Risk-sharing pools are designed to ensure that all individuals have the opportunity to purchase adequate health insurance regardless of preexisting conditions such as cancer. State laws require major insurers to participate in the plan and share the risks. Risk pools usually provide a comprehensive package of benefits with a choice of deductibles. Although the premiums are higher than individual insurance, most states impose a cap on the amount that can be charged. Some states have a waiting period for individuals with a preexisting condition, but will waive the waiting period through payment of a premium surcharge.

CONCLUSION

With the passage of the Americans With Disabilities Act of 1990, cancer survivors have an adequate base of legal remedies to combat job discrimination. The existence of legal remedies alone, however, will not prohibit future cancer-based employment discrimination. With better employer and employee education, instances of discrimination can be decreased. When discrimination does occur, survivors, as well as health and legal professionals, need to be aware of the most appropriate legal remedy, as well as constructive alternatives to a legal response. In recent years, several young adult survivors (including Ray Ritchie) have filed state and federal lawsuits upon rejection from jobs for which they were qualified. These cases can provide remedies not only for the individual plaintiffs, but, perhaps more important, discourage other employers from engaging in discriminatory practices.

Unfortunately, survivors have far fewer remedies with which to overcome barriers to health insurance. With the exception of a few state and federal laws, survivors have no legal right to adequate, affordable health insurance. New laws, including major reforms in the American health insurance system, are needed to ensure that survivors are able to obtain, keep, and enforce health insurance policies sufficient to meet their legitimate medical needs.

A more extensive discussion of this topic can be found in "Taking Care of Business: Employment, Insurance, and Money Matters." In Mullan F, Hoffman B (eds): "Charting the Journey: An Almanac of Practical Resources for the Cancer Survivor," Consumer Reports Book, Mount Vernon, 1990.

REFERENCES

1. American Cancer Society: "Facts and Figures 1990."
2. 100th Congress. 1st Session 28:1987. "Hearing on Discrimination Against Cancer Victims and the Handicapped: Hearing on HR 192 and HR 1546." Before the Subcommittee on Employment Opportunities of the House Commission on Education and Labor. (Statement of Representative Mario Biaggi, 31–33 and statement of Barbara Hoffman, National Coalition for Cancer Survivorship 41–53).

3. Feldman F: Work and Cancer Health Histories: Work Expectations and Experiences of Youth With Cancer Histories. (Ages 13–23). Report of the American Cancer Society, Oakland, California Division, 1982.

4. Wasserman AL, Thompson ET, Wilmas JA, Fairclough DL: The psychosocial status of survivors of childhood/adolescent Hodgkin's disease. Am J Dis Child 141:626–631, 1987.

5. Koocher GP, O'Malley JE: The Damocles Syndrome: Psychosocial Consequences of Surviving Childhood Cancer. New York: McGraw-Hill, 1982. Feldman F: Work and Cancer Health Histories: Work expectations and Experiences of Youth With Cancer Histories. Ages 13–23. Report of the American Cancer Society, Oakland, California Division. Fobair P, Hoppe RT, Bloom J, Cox J, Varghese A, Spiegel D: Psychosocial problems among survivors of Hodgkin's disease. J Clin Oncol 4(5): 805–814, 1986.

6. Greenleigh Associates: Report on the social, economic and psychological needs of cancer patients in California. Report of American Cancer Society, San Francisco, California Division, p 24, 1979. Also in Proceedings of Western States Conference on Cancer Rehabilitation, San Francisco, CA, 1982.

7. Teta MJ, Del Po MC, Kasl SV, Meigs JW, Myers MH, Mulvihill JJ: Psychosocial consequences of childhood and adolescent cancer survival. J Chronic Dis 39(9):751–759, 1986.

8. Rehabilitation Act of 1973: Section 2–504, 29 U.S.C. Sections 701–796i, 1986.

9. S. Rep. No. 318: 93rd Congress. 1st Session 26. Reprinted in: 1973 U.S. Code Cong. and Ad News 2076, 2092.

10. 29 U.S.C. 794, 1986.

11. 29. U.S.C. 706 (7) (B), 1986.

12. 41 C.F.R. Section 60–741.54. App A, 1984 (Emphasis Added).

13. Ritchie v City of Houston: H 87–504, ;slip op (S.D. Tex, September 2, 1988).

14. Slip Op. at 2.

15. Slip Op. at 3

16. Slip Op. at 3

17. Slip Op at 4.

18. E.g. CAL Government Code. Section 12940 (Deering 1985), VT. Stat Ann. Tit 21, Section 495d (7) (c), 1986.

19. Fla Stat Ann 760.22 (1984); Iowa Civil Rights Commission Rules 6.1(5), FEPM 453:3101 (1979); La Rev. Stat Ann 46:2253 (1982); Md. Anti-Discrimination Regulations 14.03(c), FEPM 455:717 (1979); Ann Laws of Mass 151B Section 1(17) 1985; M.S.A. 363.01 (25) (1984); N.M.S. Ann 28-1-2(k) (1983); N.Y. Exec. Law 292(21) (1984); Okla. Stat. Tit. 25, Section 1301(4) (1984); Or. Rev. Stat 659.400 (2) (1981); Pa. Human Relations Commission Handicap Discrimination Guidelines, 16 Pa. Code 44.4(d), FEPM 457:863 (1978); R.I. General Laws 28-5-6(H) (1984); Vt. Stat. Ann. Tit. 21, Section 495(d) (7) (1982); Wash. Adm Code 162-22-040(b) (iii); FEPM 457–2941 (1975); and Wis. Stat. Ann 11.32(8) (1984).

20. Chrysler Outboard Corporation v Department of Industry, Labor and Human Relations. 14 Fair Emp. Prac. Dec (CCH) at 14,9405.

21. Crothers HM: Employment problems of cancer survivors: Local problems and local solutions. In American Cancer Society: Proceedings of the Workshop on Employment, Insurance and the Patient with Cancer. American Cancer Society, New Orleans, Louisianna Division, 1986, pp 51–57.

22. Burton L and Zones J: The incidence of insurance barriers and employment discrimination among Californians with a cancer health history in 1983: A projection. American Cancer Society, Oakland, California Division, 1982.

23. National Health Policy Forum Issue Brief. No 545, May 24, 1990, Washington, DC.

24. Consolidated Omnibus Budget Reconciliation Act. 42 U.S.C. 300bb et seq (1986).

25. 29 U.S.C. 1001 et seq (1974).

26. See Vogel: Containing Medical and Disability Costs by Cutting Unhealthy Employees: Does Section 510 of ERISA Provide a Remedy? 62 Notre Dame Law. 1024 (1987).

21

Employment Problems and Workplace Experience of Childhood Cancer Survivors

Daniel M. Hays, M.D., John Landsverk, Ph.D., Kathleen Ruccione, R.N., M.P.H., Diana Schoonover, B.A., Susan L. Zilber, M.Phil., and Stuart E. Siegel, M.D.

As a result of the therapeutic advances made during the past three decades, the majority of children in the United States afflicted with cancer will now survive to join the workforce. As survival in this group of individuals may be measured in decades rather than years, the total number of childhood cancer survivors is at present rapidly increasing. This preliminary report analyzes the long-range employment experience of adults who are childhood cancer survivors and were treated at a single institution, Childrens Hospital Los Angeles (CHLA). Subsequent studies will combine data from two additional pediatric centers and include a younger age group.

MATERIALS AND METHODS

Eligible for entry into the study were surviving patients treated for cancer at CHLA during the years 1942–1985, who were 20 or more years of age in 1988. In all cases, the diagnosis of cancer was made prior to the patient's nineteenth birthday, and all patients were disease-free for a minimum of two years after the end of therapy. In addition, all of the well-recognized categories of malignant tumors of childhood (Table 1), the study group included survivors of all types of central nervous system (CNS) tumors, irrespec-

tive of histology, and children with several tumors of questionable malignancy who received therapy for cancer.

Potential survivors were traced through hospital records, voters' registration and tax lists, death certificates, bride/groom indices, motor vehicle registration, and credit bureaus. Death was established in 535 former patients. Telephone contact was made with 368 survivors and 358 of these were interviewed. Seven (2%) refused to be interviewed, and 23 (6%) of the interviews were by "proxy." In the latter cases, information was provided by relatives. This group had permanent major disability (17 subjects) or were shielded from contact by parents (six subjects). Subjects with proxy interviews were regarded as "disabled" by the interviewed relative (80%), on permanent public assistance (85%), and less than 25% of these survivors were concerned with vocational opportunities. Diagnoses in these cases were CNS tumors, bilateral retinoblastoma, post-cardiac arrest syndrome, and other major complications of management. As their problems were unique, this group (constituting 6% of all survivors) was not included in subsequent analyses, except as indicated.

A basic interview instrument of 356 items was administered to survivors by telephone at a time convenient to the subject. Interviews were conducted by professional health science interviewers and were carried out largely during evening and weekend hours. Mean duration of subject interviews was 69.9 (SD 38.6) min, and the majority were carried out by three individuals. Controls were selected from a panel of up to six individuals provided by the survivor. Same-sex siblings within two years of the age of the subject were preferred. Each potential control was evaluated by a five minute "preliminary" interview by telephone, and following analysis of the information obtained from these, the closest "match" was selected for the final control interview. Controls with a history of cancer were excluded. Emphasis in matching was placed on factors known to influence economic status, particularly the educational and economic achievement of each parent, with sex, age, and race additional factors. Of the 627 potential controls, 335 were individually matched to 335 subjects. Fifteen potential controls refused to be interviewed and were replaced. In the interview instrument for controls, the term "cancer" was replaced by "any health problem" in items that referred to specific factors associated with cancer or its therapy. There were no controls for the patients with proxy interviews.

Medical records of subjects were abstracted, including surgical, radiotherapy, and chemotherapy variables. Information regarding subjects was supplemented during routine visits to the Long-Range Oncology Clinic (1987–1990). Prior to or following the telephone interviews, 36 of the interviewed survivors were seen here, the history was reviewed, physical examination carried out, and appropriate laboratory or roentgenographic studies performed. These clinic visits corroborated responses made during interviews, but provided little additional information in socioeconomic areas. Data from the subject interviews, control interviews, and medical record abstractions were entered for analysis. Differences between groups on discrete variables were calculated by chi-square tests and continuous variables by Student's t-tests.

RESULTS

Pathologic diagnoses among the 358 survivors interviewed, including the 335 matched-pair group, are listed in Table 1. Among those survivors 30 years of age and older, the most frequent diagnosis was nephroblastoma (Wilms' tumor) followed by CNS tumors. Among survivors from the next cohort, now 20–29 years of age, leukemia had assumed a dominant position as a most frequent diagnosis among survivors. The mean age at diagnosis was 7.7 years (SD 5.3) (range < 1–18 years) and the mean interval between diagnosis and entry into the study was 19.0 years (SD 8.4) (range 4–39 years).

A survivor versus control comparison, including the 335 matched pairs (Table 2), showed no significant differences in racial/ethnic background, educational achievements of parents, or Duncan Socioeconomic Indices for parents. The controls were same-sex siblings within two years of the age of the subjects in 34.4% of the matched pairs.

The lifelong employment experience of the survivors and controls, in respect both to obtaining positions and their subsequent relations with employers and co-workers, are summarized in Table 3. In item number 1 (Table 3), the responses of subject versus control groups are not comparable, as subjects were referring only to their history of cancer in their response, while controls might include reference to any health problem. Among the comparisons that were significant, a higher proportion of the subjects felt that, at some time, they were denied a position for which they believed they were qualified,

TABLE 1. Childhood Cancer Survivors: Diagnoses

| | Age at time of interview | | | | | |
	>30 years	(%)	20–29 years	(%)	Total	(%)
Leukemia	6	(5)	54	(22)	60	(17)
Nephroblastoma	22	(20)	33	(13)	55	(15)
Central nervous system	21	(19)	26	(10)	47	(13)
Hodgkin's disease	8	(7)	32	(13)	40	(11)
Neuroblastoma	10	(9)	11	(4)	21	(6)
Histiocytosis	12	(11)	8	(3)	20	(6)
Non-Hodgkin's lymphoma	1	(1)	16	(6)	17	(5)
Other solid tumors	30	(27)	68	(27)	98	(27)
Total	**110**		**248**		**358**[a]	

[a]Includes 23 survivors interviewed "by proxy."

and 34.6% of the survivors believed that this denial was related to their cancer history. The percentage of survivors who had been denied entry into one of the Armed Services was significantly greater than controls and almost entirely attributed by survivors to their history of cancer. Social discrimination by co-workers was also more common among survivors (Item 6, Table 3). In Item 7 (Table 3), again, a direct comparison is not possible. This item concerned the situation in which the survivor did not make a possibly advantageous change in employment because of concerns regarding: a) the influence of his/her cancer history on the new job situation; or b) the insurance related effects of such a move. In respect to controls, this was a broader question concerning reasons, health-related or otherwise, for re-

TABLE 2. Survivor-Control Matched Pairs (335 Pairs)

	Subjects		Controls	
Male subjects and controls	50.1%		50.1%	
Female subjects and controls	49.9%		49.9%	
Age at interview	26.7 years		27.5 years	
	(5.9)[a]		(6.0)	
Same-sex sibling				
(<2 years age difference)		34.4%		
Race/ethnicity				
Non-Hispanic white	70.3%		74.0%	
Hispanic	18.0%		19.4%	
Black	3.9%		2.1%	
Asian/Others	7.8%		0.5%	
Highest school grade completed (years)				
Father of subject/control	13.1	(3.4)	13.3	(3.2)
Mother of subject/control	12.7	(2.9)	13.0	(2.6)
Duncan Socioeconomic Index (DSEI)				
Father of subject/control	46.6	(24.2)	48.3	(24.6)
Mother of subject/control	44.7	(20.3)	45.8	(21.2)

[a]SD from the mean.

TABLE 3. Employment History of Survivors/Controls (335 Matched Pairs)

	Subjects (%)	Controls (%)	P
1. Always revealed cancer (health) history to potential employer?	43.5	63.8	
2. Ever denied job for which you were qualified?	31.5 (34.6)[a]	24.5	0.04
3. Ever denied a promotion when qualified?	17.5 (15.5)	15.8	NS
4. Ever denied entry into armed services?	11.3 (94.7)	4.5	0.001
5. Ever denied job in police/fire departments?	2.7 (33.3)	2.4	NS
6. Ever noted discrimination by co-workers At work? Socially?	3.3 6.6	1.5 1.8	NS 0.002
7. Ever rejected an alternative and possibly more rewarding job opportunity because of their cancer history/health history?	4.8	17.1	

[a]The number in parentheses represents the proportion of the percent above it that was attributed by the survivors to their history of cancer. NS, significant.

luctance to make a change to a possibly more satisfactory position.

The employment status of survivors and controls at the time of the interview (1987–1989) is detailed in Table 4. The first five items were responses to the inquiry "Which of these describes your life now?" with the eight (condensed to five) listed by the interviewer. Among subjects, 7.8% regarded themselves as "disabled" (item 1, Table 4) versus 2.1% of controls. This did not preclude those who considered themselves as "disabled" from having full-time employment and health insurance. The Duncan Socioeconomic Index [1,2], an established system of rating employment positions of all types on the basis of remuneration and the length of training (or education) required was similar in both groups. Remaining items in Table 4 were not mutually exclusive. Many of those currently working were also students, particularly those in part-time work status. Those who were self-employed were also included in item 1, Table 4 as "currently working."

Table 5 summarizes a large group of items related to the history of workplace activities of survivors and controls. In respect to having missed workdays without permission, conflicts with supervisors, disciplinary actions, and termination of employment, the subjects and controls were similar. Survivors asked for special provisions in the workplace less frequently than controls. The size of the workforce in the companies or businesses in which survivors and controls worked was divided into six categories. The distribution of survivors was comparable to that of the controls, that is, survivors were not found more frequently in institutions with a large work force.

DISCUSSION

Discrimination in employment and other problems among survivors of adult

TABLE 4. Present Employment and Educational Status

	Subjects (%)	Controls (%)	P
1. Currently			
Working, full-time or part-time?[a]	78.8	81.2	NS
Unemployed, looking for work?	8.0	5.6	NS
Unemployed, not looking for work?	6.8	5.3	NS
Keeping house?	21.5	19.1	NS
"Disabled"?	7.8	2.1	< 0.001
2. Duncan SEI Index	44.3	46.7	NS
3. Currently working at usual job?	67.4	69.5	NS
4. Present job is commensurate with the subject's/control's skills?	68.8	68.8	NS
5. Self-employed?	10.3	9.0	NS
6. Currently a student?	25.1	20.9	NS
7. Highest school grade (completed years)	13.8 (SD ± 1.9)	13.9 (SD ± 2.0)	NS

[a]Responses to this question are not mutually exclusive. NS, not significant.

forms of cancer has been subjected to intensive study for four decades. Important differences between the survivors of adult forms of cancer and the survivors of childhood cancer include: a) the frequently extended period of survival before entering the workforce in the case of the latter; and b) the lack of a prior employment record or of established skills among many childhood survivors. An initial study of childhood cancer survivors by Feldman in 1980 [3] included 200 interviews with survivors, parents, physicians, teachers, and employers relative to discrimination in the workplace observed in Los Angeles during the 1960s and early 1970s. She noted that 45% of the adult survivors of childhood cancer had been denied employment because of a history of cancer. Reflecting the lack of legal concerns of that era, in 75% of these cases a cancer-related basis for this denial was confirmed by the employer involved. Feldman observed a trend towards "job stability" among child-

TABLE 5. History of Workplace Activities: Survivors/Controls

	Subjects (%)	Controls (%)	P
1. Work days missed during the past year?	75.0	73.0	NS
2. Conflicts with supervisor regarding work assignment during past year?	5.1	7.8	NS
3. Disciplinary actions by employer during past year?	6.5	6.0	NS
4. Ever "fired" or "laid off"?	34.5	32.9	NS
5. Ever asked for special provisions in the workplace for health reasons?	10.3	14.8	NS

NS, not significant.

hood cancer survivors once employed and the reluctance of the pediatric cancer survivor to admit work-related or other limitations. In a similar interview study by Koocher and O'Malley (1981) [4], the initial rejection rate for employment by work-able youth was 25%. A study by Phillips, Pizzo, and Gerber in 1985 [5], of 83 pediatric cancer survivors with partial sibling controls showed 81% of the subjects were employed, but among pairs of matched siblings, in 12 among 25 pairs the annual income of the survivor was substantially lower than that of the control ($P < 0.03$).

Teta et al. in 1986 [6], after interviews with 450 childhood cancer survivors and 587 sibling controls, noted discrimination relative to entering the uniformed services and in the workplace situation for males but not females. Fobair et al. in 1986 [7] found the rate of problems associated with employment to be 42% among young adults with Hodgkin's disease, who were interviewed 10 years following the end of therapy. Eighteen percent of males and 42% of females were described as "unemployed" at the time of the interview. Problems in the employment area were concentrated in patients with advanced disease (Stages III or IV) and among those who received maximum amounts of chemotherapy as opposed to combined therapy [8].

Kelaghan et al. in 1988 [9] noted that educational achievement was reduced among survivors of therapy for CNS tumors, but not among other cancer survivors. Tebbi et al. in 1989 [10] conducted a study of the long-term vocational achievement of 40 survivors in whom cancer was recognized during adolescence and found that 7.4% reported disease-related discrimination during the hiring process and 66.7% relative to induction into the military. In a study of 95 younger survivors (mean age, 23.6 years; median age, 22 years) by Meadows et al. in 1989 [11],

13.7% were unemployed and only 52.96% had full-time employment. An employment rate of 73% was found among 227 young survivors responding to a questionnaire by Green et al. in 1990 [12]. Most of these studies have been summarized by Crothers [13].

In the present study, educational achievement was almost identical in survivor and control groups. The lifetime history of some survivors (although not a majority of survivors in this study) reveals evidence of discrimination (some blatant) in many of the areas associated with employment. This was particularly evident during the period 1943–1975, that is, among the older survivors. It should be noted that the National Rehabilitation Act was enacted in 1973 and the Fair Employment Practice Act (California) in 1974, both of which were designed to eliminate (among other things) discrimination in employment on the basis of a history of cancer. Although only one of the survivors in the present study has instituted legal/administrative action on the basis of discrimination and despite the impression of most observers that childhood cancer survivors are generally reticent to initiate legal action, the effect of these legislative efforts on the attitudes of employers has probably been significant.

The most powerful predictors of ultimate economic status for the individual U.S. resident are the educational and economic achievements of parents, and this weighed heavily in the selection of controls. We employed the Duncan Socioeconomic Index [2] as the most sensitive measure of economic status, and the difference between subject and control groups relative to this measure was not significant.

The mean age of survivors in the CHLA series presented here is approximately 27 years. The majority have surmounted problems in employment discrimination and now have workplace situations that are as acceptable to them as are the comparable situations of their controls. Their "job" categories are similar to controls. In regard to a broad group of potential problems occurring in the workplace, the survivors and controls are similar in every respect.

There are several areas of significant difference between survivors and controls. Among survivors, 7.8% regarded themselves as "disabled" versus 2.1% of the controls. These were not subjects with proxy interviews, and in both the subject and control groups almost all of these individuals had full-time employment and health insurance. This would appear, then, to represent a perception of social rather than economic status, which was also suggested by Item 6, Table 3. Although discrimination in respect to positions in police and fire departments was not demonstrated, entry into all branches of the armed services was clearly difficult for survivors.

Advisors to survivors have stressed the advantage of employment opportunities in large companies, in which the employment policies are relatively "open," but despite such advice, there was no concentration of survivors in large businesses or institutions as opposed to the control group.

Several investigators recognized a "severe late-effects" group (Greenberg et al., 1989) [14], or emphasized the psychosocial problems of special subgroups of survivors with physical defects [15,16,17]. The "impaired" survivor group in the present study includes patients demonstrating the effects of CNS tumors and/or their therapy, major amputations, blindness and, to a lesser extent, intestinal or urinary stomas. However, not _all_ survivors in any of these categories could be assigned to this group. In prior studies, many survivors in this impaired group have histories of poor academic achievement, "loss of friends" [15], and employment problems.

As they leave the childhood and adolescent periods, these survivors continue to need "age-specific" active and adaptable rehabilitation in its broadest sense. The percentage of childhood cancer survivors in this group was placed as high as 22% by Greenberg et al., [14], but in the present series was approximately 5%.

This preliminary report presents a small part of the data, which will be available from this study, on the employment problems of the childhood cancer survivor. It suggests that, in many respects, the survivors' problems are less general then they were in the 1960s and 1970s, and that interventions need to be more narrowly focused on specific problems for different categories of survivors.

ACKNOWLEDGMENTS

This study was supported by USPHS grants CA-44133 and CA-23146 awarded by the National Cancer Institute, National Institutes of Health, Bethesda, Maryland.

REFERENCES

1. McTavish D: A method for more reliably coding detailed occupations into Duncan's socioeconomic categories. Am Soc Rev 29:402–406, 1964.
2. Blau PM, Duncan OW (eds): The American Occupational Structure. New York: Wiley, 1967.
3. Feldman FL: Work and Cancer Health Histories: Work Expectations and Experiences of Youth with Cancer Histories (Ages 13–23). Summary Report. Oakland CA: American Cancer Society (California Division), 1980.
4. Koocher GP, O'Malley JE (ed): The Damocles Syndrome: Psychosocial Consequences of Surviving Childhood Cancer. New York: McGraw-Hill Book Co, 1981.
5. Phillips S, Pizzo P, Gerber L: Work status of childhood cancer survivors. (Abstract). Childhood Cancer Survivors: Living beyond cure. Tenth Annual Mental Health Conference, April 11–12, 1985, Houston, TX, 1985.
6. Teta MJ, Del Po MC, Kase SV, et al.: Psychosocial consequences of childhood and adolescent cancer survival. J Chronic Dis 39:751–759, 1986.

7. Fobair P, Hoppe RT, Bloom J et al.: Psychosocial problems among survivors of Hodgkin's disease. J Clin Oncol 4:805–814, 1986.

8. Cella DF, Tross S: Psychological adjustment to survival from Hodgkin's disease. J Cons Clin Psychol 54:616–622, 1986.

9. Kelaghan J, Myers MH, Mulvihill JJ, et al.: Educational achievement of long-term survivors of childhood and adolescent cancer. Med Pediatr Oncol 16:320–326, 1988.

10. Tebbi CK, Bromberg C, Piedmonte M: Long-term vocational adjustment of cancer patients diagnosed during adolescence. Cancer 63:213–218, 1989.

11. Meadows AT, McKee L, Kazak AE: Psychosocial status of young adult survivors of childhood cancer: A survey. Med Pediatr Oncol 17:466–470, 1989.

12. Green D, Zevon M, Hall B: Achievement of life goals by adult survivors of modern treatment for childhood cancer. Cancer 67:206–213, 1991.

13. Crothers HM: Employment problems of cancer survivors: Local problems and local solutions. Proceedings of the Workshop on Employment, Insurance and the Patient with Cancer. American Cancer Society, New Orleans, 1987.

14. Greenberg HS, Kazak AE, Meadows AT: Psychologic functioning in 8- to 16-year old cancer survivors and their parents. J Pediatr 114:488–493, 1989.

15. Tebbi CK, Mallon JC: Long-term psychosocial outcome among cancer amputees in adolescence and early adulthood. J Psy Oncol 5:69–82, 1987.

16. Ganz PA: Current issues in cancer rehabilitation. Cancer 65:742–751, 1990.

17. Tebbi CK, Stern M, et al.: The role of social support systems in adolescent cancer amputees. Cancer 56:965–971, 1985.

22

Long-Term Survivors: Empowerment for the Twenty-First Century

Grace Powers Monaco, J.D.

Survivors of pediatric cancer have often been exposed to radiation and to an overwhelming panoply of chemotherapeutic agents. They, therefore, have special sensitivities and potential organ system problems. These necessarily influence the choice of procedures and drugs required to test complications or unrelated conditions that might develop later in life. These include: cardiac dysfunctions, musculoskeletal, thyroid, and immunologic abnormalities, neurophysiological difficulties, benign and malignant neoplasms, and psychosocial sequelae [1,2].

Complete and accurate data on these susceptibilities and on genetic predispositions for the survivors and their families are needed so that new, less toxic, and more effective therapies can be refined and tailored to risks [1,2,13–17].

Most pediatric cancer patients have a general awareness that they may be at risk in a variety of ways from their disease and its treatment. However, as they mature, move away from home, go to college, pursue careers, and make important changes in their lives, the responsibility for health care comes to rest on them and not their parents.

At present, the adult former child patient often does not appreciate how vital his/her past medical history can be. These young adults may not understand that, when they develop some medical problem, it is important that the physician knows that they received X treatment as a child. A sign or symptom may have special implications because of their unusual medical history. And without assistance, they surely will not remember what types of chemotherapy and procedures they had, and/or where they had them [1,18].

The current practice of insurers to refuse to provide life, health, and disability insurance to many childhood cancer survivors fosters the wish or need to hide the past [19–22].

Physicians who treat these patients may be internists and general practitioners who, because they are called upon infrequently to treat cancer survivors, may not have a working knowledge of recent medical developments (e.g., what to watch out for, what to avoid, and what to report to the original treatment center).

Candlelighters' Childhood Cancer Foundation (CCCF) is cooperating in a grant proposal that will facilitate networking among long-term care clinics, extend the benefits of access to targeted follow-up services, and provide an easily accessible data base for researchers to use in following survivors and pediatric cancer families.

This grant proposal was built particularly on the wisdom of Dr. A. Meadows and Dr. G. D'Angio's call for preparation of our survivors for being the in-charge unit for lifetime medical surveillance [1,13,22,33]. It builds upon the collabora-

Late Effects of Treatment for Childhood Cancer, pages 179–182 © 1992 Wiley-Liss, Inc.

tive relationship among family–patient–care giver that has been the hallmark of the pediatric cancer experience, and carries that relationship into the age of survivorship.

Building blocks include the family and peer support program of CCCF and the services of late effects clinics and treatment facilities. A decline in available social support is presently noted for survivors of childhood cancer [35]. The proposed "locator" service would help to address this need while at the same time maximizing follow-up of patients for epidemiological and biostatistical data [22–26]. The competence to address this problem is already in place [22–32,34].

The Treatment Center has proven that it can successfully educate families and patients to a wide variety of self-care and advocacy tasks. The Treatment Center has established that it can also be a unit of advocacy, particularly in insurance, employment, and education outreach.

The Medical Care Team/Parent collaboration on surveillance, interventions, and rehabilitation has been successful in promoting the truly whole personhood of the survivor and family.

Studies have documented that patient compliance is enhanced and outcomes improved when the patient/family is involved in a strong supportive network: family and/or peer [25,35].

DEVELOPMENT OF A NATIONAL NETWORKING PROGRAM FOR SURVIVORS

Building upon what we have learned from the parent, center, and late effects clinic follow-up experience, a networking program with newsletters, opportunities for advocacy, and personal contact/groups as needed, will keep survivors "in touch" up close or at a distance (as they desire).

Chesler's survey [18] demonstrated that our survivors want to be in touch and want to "help" younger survivors make it. This also would help address the decline in available social support for survivors who have "left" the treatment system. Workshops were held at CCCF 20th anniversary conference in Washington in July 1990 to address survivor needs and initiate networking opportunities. The Adult Survivors of Childhood Cancer Network, with technical assistance from CCCF, has begun special publications for "youth" with cancer, self-help guides, and an ombudsman program assisting in insurance and employment problems.

The network will facilitate development of a model treatment center education program to train survivors to be empowered medical consumers, knowledgable about the need for continued medical surveillance, and advocates for themselves and each other.

The network will participate in the development of a "locator" service with "personalized coded card" and possibly personal copies on disc for physician/patient access to complete medical records including a protocol for follow-up and history, and sensitivities. Records would be available through computer access for fax, and provision will be made for update via direct computer entry to the centralized source or treatment center by fax.

The work carried out under submitted grants would determine the most feasible mechanism to provide the survivors with: a) their own "portable" and regularly updated medical records, and b) a private code that would permit their physician(s) direct access to the central (or decentralized) computer systems containing the permanent storage of these records. We are investing the "graduate" of cancer treatment with a very special type of empowerment and control [27,31].

Survivor access to records and control over future medical care fits one of the primary goals for childhood cancer patients and survivors—to "take charge of their lives" [18,22,36–38]. This provides the opportunity to break free from the period of dependency on parents, which is extended because of their cancer [36–38].

The "graduates" will be provided with access to peers directly or through publications; to education, information, opportunities for advocacy participation and counseling of younger patients and to the most up-to-date medical, psychosocial, political, legal, educational, and employment impact information. All of this will enhance their skills for adult survival and, in fact, through their own unique "old boys network," provide some advantages in networking for success in their lives.

REFERENCES

1. D'Angio G: Cure is not enough: Late consequences associated with radiation treatment. J Assoc Ped Oncol Nurses 5(4):20–23, 1988.
2. Lange BJ, Meadows AT: Late effects of Hodgkin's disease treatments in children. Cancer Treat Rep 41:195–220, 1989.
3. Moshang T Jr, Lee MM: Late effects: Disorders of growth and sexual maturation associated with the treatment of childhood cancer. J Assoc Pediatr Oncol Nurses 5(4):14–19, 1988.
4. Peckham VC: Learning disorders associated with the treatment of cancer in childhood. J Assoc Pediatr Oncol Nurses 5(4):10–13, 1988.
5. Pfefferbaum-Levine B et al.: Neuropsychologic assessment of long-term survivors of childhood leukemia. Am J Pediatr Hematol Oncol 6(2):123–127, 1984.
6. Williams JA, Thompson EI: Results of therapy for Hodgkin's disease at St. Jude Children's Research Hospital. Cancer Treat Rep 41:303–306, 1989.
7. Fobair P et al.: Psychosocial problems among survivors of Hodgkin's disease. J Clin Oncol 4:806–814, 1986.
8. Teta MJ et al.: Psychosocial consequences of childhood and adolescent cancer survival. J Chron Dis 39(9):751–759, 1986.
9. Duffner PK, Cohen ME, Parker MS: Prospective intellectual testing in children with brain tumors. Annals Neurol 23(6):575–579, 1988.
10. Meadows AT et al.: Second malignant neoplasms in children: An update from the Late Effects Study Group. J Clin Oncol 3(4):532–538, 1985.
11. Meadows A: Learning problems associated with therapy for acute lymphocytic leukemia (ALL). Candlelighters' Childhood Cancer Foundation Progress Report IV93:11–12, 1984.
12. Meadows AT, Kreymas NL, Belasco JB: The medical cost of cure: Sequelae in survivors of childhood cancer. In van Eys J, Sullivan MP (eds): Status of the Curability of Childhood Cancer. New York: Raven Press, 1980, pp 263–276.
13. Meadows AT: The concept of care of life. J Assoc Pediatr Oncol Nurses 5(4):7–9, 1988.
14. Polednak AP: Survival of children diagnosed with acute lymphoblastic leukemia in 1977–1981 in Connecticut. J Clin Epidemiol 42(7):617–623, 1985.
15. Greenberg RS, Shuster JL Jr: Epidemiology of cancer in children. Epidemiol Rev 7:22–28, 1985.
16. Hass JE, Muczynski KA, Krailo M, Ablin A, Land V, Vietti TJ, Hammond GD: Histopathology and prognosis in childhood hepatoblastoma and hepatocarcinoma. Cancer 64(5):1082–1085, 1989.
17. Mulvihill JJ, Connelly RR, et al: Cancer in offspring of long-term survivors of childhood and adolescent cancer. Lancet ii: 813–817, 1987.
18. Chesler M, Lozowski S: Problems and needs of children off treatment: Candlelighters' research and proposed programs. Candlelighters' Childhood Cancer Foundation Quarterly Newsletter XII:2–3, 1989.
19. Feldman FL: Work and cancer health histories: Work expectations and experiences of youth with cancer histories (Ages 13–23). American Cancer Society, California Division, Oakland, CA, 1980.
20. Holmes GE et al.: The availability of insurance to long time survivors of childhood cancer. Cancer 57:190–193, 1986.
21. Monaco GP: CCCF advocacy series: Your insurance and your child's. 1989.
22. Monaco GP: Socioeconomic considerations in childhood cancer survival: Society's obligations. Childhood Cancer Survivors: Living beyond Cure. Am J Pediatr Hematol 9(1):92–98, 1987.
23. McCalla JL: A multidisciplinary approach to identification and remedial intervention for adverse late effects of cancer therapy. Nursing Clinics of North America 20(1):117–129, 1985.
24. Barofsky I: Therapeutic compliance and the cancer patient. Health Educ Q (Special Suppl) 10:43–56, 1984.
25. Monaco GP: Parent self-help groups families of children with cancer. Ca-A Cancer J Clin 38:41–47, 1988.

26. Chesler M and Barbarin OA: Childhood cancer and the family. New York: Bruner-Mazel, 1987.

27. Greenfield S, Kaplan S, Ware J: Expanding patient involvement in care: Effects on patient outcomes. Ann Int Med 102:520–528, 1985.

28. Heiney SP, Ruffin J, Ettinger R, Ettinger S: The effects of group therapy on adolescents with cancer. J Assoc Ped Oncol Nurses 1(4):16, 1984.

29. Kieffer C: Citizens empowerment: A developmental perspective. Prev Human Sev 3(2/3):9–36, 1983–1984.

30. Nathanson MN: Organizing and maintaining support groups for parents of children with chronic illness and handicapping conditions. Association for the Care of Children's Health, Washington, DC, 1986.

31. Nathanson MN, Monaco GP: Meeting the educational and psychosocial needs produced by a diagnosis of pediatric/adolescent cancer. Cancer Patient Educ, Health Educ Qu (Special Suppl) 10:67–75, 1984.

32. Patient Booklet. Center for Cancer Treatment and Research. Richland Memorial Hospital, 1988.

33. Rappaport J: Studies in empowerment. Prev Human Serv 3(2/3):1–8, 1983–1984.

34. Yoak M, Chesney B, Schwartz N: Active roles in self-help groups for parents of children with cancer. Children's Health Care 14(1):38–40, 1985.

35. Deasy-Spinetta P: CCCF: Private consultation on need for educational intervention beyond reentry for children with cancer, 1987.

36. Byrne CM, Stockwell M, Gudelis S: Adolescent support groups in oncology. ONF 11(4):36, 1984.

37. Holmes HA, Holmes FF: After ten years what are the handicaps and lifestyles of children treated for cancer. Am Pediatr 14:819–823, 1985.

38. Young MA, Pfefferbaum-Levine B: Perspectives on illness and treatment in adolescence. Cancer Bull 36(6):275, 1984.

Index